Developing Expertise in Critical Care Nursing

Julie Scholes

With contributions from

John Albarran and Caroline Williams

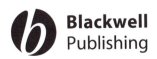

Blackwell
Publishing

Blackwell Publishing editorial offices:
Blackwell Publishing Ltd, 9600 Garsington Road, Oxford OX4 2DQ, UK
    Tel: +44 (0)1865 776868
Blackwell Publishing Inc., 350 Main Street, Malden, MA 02148-5020, USA
    Tel: +1 781 388 8250
Blackwell Publishing Asia Pty Ltd, 550 Swanston Street, Carlton, Victoria 3053, Australia
    Tel: +61 (0)3 8359 1011

First published 2006 by Blackwell Publishing Ltd

ISBN-10: 1-4051-1715-X
ISBN-13: 978-1-4051-1715-9

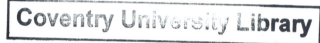

Library of Congress Cataloging-in-Publication Data
Scholes, Julie.
Developing expertise in critical care nursing/Julie Scholes; with contributions from John Albarran and Caroline Williams.
      p. ; cm.
   Includes bibliographical references and index.
   ISBN-13: 978-1-4051-1715-9 (pbk. : alk. paper)
   ISBN-10: 1-4051-1715-X (pbk. : alk. paper)
   1. Intensive care nursing.   2. Nursing diagnosis.   I. Albarran, John W.   II. Williams, Caroline, 1963–   III. Title.
   [DNLM: 1. Critical Care–organization & administration.   2. Critical Illness–nursing.
   3. Nursing Care–organization & administration.   WY 154 S368d 2006]
RT120.I5S36 2006
610.73'6–dc22
2006008651

A catalogue record for this title is available from the British Library

Set in 10/12.5pt Palatino
by Graphicraft Limited, Hong Kong
Printed and bound in India
by Replika Press Pvt Ltd, Kundli

For further information on Blackwell Publishing, visit our website:
www.blackwellpublishing.com

In memory of Alan Boylan and Di Moore, inspirational nurse teachers, whose passion and commitment to the profession were a constant source of motivation, joy and energy.
I hope this book does our conversations justice.

To Dad, who taught me that tenacity and determination will get you through any transition, especially when served with a large portion of humour and humility.

Contents

Foreword

Transitions are an inevitable dimension of many aspects of our lives, a product perhaps of contemporary approaches to life! This innovative text is designed to assist critical care nurses through one of the most important transitions – how we move, and assist others to move, along the continuum towards expertise. Having expertise and being able to share it are not merely two sides of the same coin and the central thesis of this text is that expertise has to be actively transmitted. It has become fashionable in certain quarters to bemoan the current state of the profession and to don rose-coloured glasses when reminiscing about how things used to be. This text reminds us that the responsibility for ensuring that the *essence* and *expertise* of nursing is passed to the next generation lies with all of us.

The three conceptual building blocks for the text (evidence, experience and reflection) are supported by the use of analogy, which assists with the grasp of key constructs. I particularly liked the notion of expertise as a graphic equaliser (p. 4) to describe different elements of expertise. However, the work moves beyond a purely theoretical approach to expertise and provides those at all points on the 'novice–expert' continuum with a repertoire of strategies to facilitate transmission of expertise, for example the toolkit on p. 218 for surviving transitions. This is also exemplified through the use of personal reflection in some of the vignettes (see Chapter 2). The marrying of this practical approach with role transition theory provides a useful bridge for the (often misunderstood) theory–practice gap.

The value of narration in the 'real world' of practice emphasised in this text provides a salient reminder of the need to retain expert clinicians at the bedside, where patients, families, students and less experienced nurses can benefit from their insights. It also reminds us of the need for experts to develop and refine their skills of narrative commentary.

This book marks a key milestone in Professor Scholes' contribution to our thinking about expert practice in critical care. Her willingness to challenge the thinking of others is a hallmark of her writing and is ably demonstrated in this text (see for example Chapter 10). Similarly, a strength of commissioned research undertaken by Scholes (and colleagues) is that they do not shirk from making clear recommendations for change, for example the need for a fifth –

acute and critical care – branch in the UK pre-registration curriculum (see p. 210).

The text draws on evidence from a number of studies undertaken in the UK. However, from an international perspective, this text has much to offer critical care nurses in all countries. Many of the vignettes will resonate and the strategies proposed will not be limited by country-specific policies and practices.

In the same way that the work of Benner and colleagues was pivotal in describing much of the 'what' and 'how' of critical care nursing (and struck a chord with so many of us), what we now need is to debate the 'how can we . . .' in order to ensure that the essence of expert critical care *nursing* continues to grow and develop. I believe this text serves this purpose. The author has wisely avoided producing lists of competencies which would otherwise tie the text to a geographical location and point in time. It is of interest, however, that at the time of publication the contribution of expert nurses in the UK is in an ambiguous position, with increasing evidence pointing to positive patient and service outcomes, yet financial constraints in the NHS leading some of these 'expensive' positions to be placed in jeopardy. This text is therefore timely and should equip critical care nurses to continue to evolve, describe and transmit their expert practice in the manner best suited to patient needs.

Professor Ruth Endacott
Professor of Critical Care Nursing
University of Plymouth, UK
La Trobe University, Australia

Preface

This book sets out to identify ways to support the development of expertise in critical care nurses. To the newcomer, critical care is a bewildering medley of lights, noise and demands that can sometimes obscure the patient and their relatives. To an expert, the visual displays and alarms assist them to engage with the patient with greater intensity and frees their conscious attention to the immediate act of caring, and decision making. This book examines the way in which a practitioner makes the transition from someone who is intellectually paralysed by all these demands to someone who demonstrates mastery of this environment, and the knowledge base to inform their practice. The ambition is to offer a repertoire of learning and assessment activities that can enable practitioners to grow their own expertise and foster developments in others. This has been presented as learning transition theory. Learning transition theory provides a generic set of skills that can be applied to the practitioner's own context, and helps them to celebrate their own professional knowledge. A menu of competencies and skills to gauge expertise is not included in this text because firstly and secondly, my argument is that expertise is so dynamic, transitory and elusive that the menu would rapidly become out of date. Other texts provide insight into the necessary scientific and professional knowledge to inform clinical competence, and readers are guided to these seminal texts if this information is required.

Critical questions are raised about the current nature of expertise within critical care practice. The central argument is that without clear facilitation of colleagues and transmission of expertise from one colleague to another, the nature of critical care nursing is at risk.

Experts in the future will face significant challenges as advances in technology and monitoring might be proffered as suitable surrogates that further distance the nurse from the patient. This would be bad for patients and their relatives as this denies the patient the importance of therapeutic human contact and does not take account of the limitations of artificial intelligence in the formulation of clinical decisions. More immediately, workforce reconfiguration, with different people working differently, demands that expert nurses find clear expression of the contribution they make to the experiences of critical care patients and their relatives. Nursing does need to grow and adapt to meet the demands of a dynamic and modernising service, but should evolve with care. The transmission of the art and science of nursing crafted by experts to realise its therapeutic potential is crucial. However, the next generation has to be receptive to the message and skills that are being passed on if they are to be assisted in their quest for expertise. This book offers strategies to address these issues.

The first task is to set out the principles on which this book is built to make clear the sources of knowledge and experience that have given this book its theoretical shape.

The argument presented in this book is that expertise is acquired through cycles of critical, facilitated reflection on experience and on evaluation of performance, which may take the form of assessment or appraisal. This leads to practice development in dynamic iterative cycles. Each spiral progressively builds and refines expertise and triggers the recognition for further development. As an outcome of each cycle it is important to share with colleagues the learning that has taken place from these iterative cycles because the articulation of experiential wisdom or aspects of expertise is crucial to stimulate others. Although the professional and academic background of the practitioner will influence the language used to express aspects of expertise, this should not obscure the nature of what is being expressed nor necessarily lead to the premature attribution of expertise.

The conceptual building blocks for the book: evidence, experience and reflection

The examination of the impact of various learning experiences on such change, or role transition at various stages in the clinical career, has been the focus for much of my research. This book has provided me with an opportunity to revisit some of this work and re-examine it in the context of contemporary critical care nursing and propose a theory of learning transitions that enable the acquisition of expertise. What unites all these studies is that data have been collected from a range of stakeholders who influenced or experienced clinical and academic learning about nursing. Importantly, all these studies involved being in the real world of clinical practice to observe first hand the impact this learning had on nurses working with their patients.

A secondary driver influenced the inception of this book. Two years ago I had a riding accident which resulted in my becoming a consumer of critical and acute care services. This was a salutary experience and a significant personal role transition from researcher used to standing beside critical care practitioners to understand and analyse what they do, to a patient, lying on a bed staring up at them experiencing the service first hand. This was an extremely powerful and painful experience. I was privileged to experience excellent care. I am reminded and humbled by the great acts of kindness and extraordinary professionalism displayed by those who helped me. I am also stunned by the memory resonance of those who did not seek to do me harm, but who did so, by a cast-off word or gesture. However, these encounters enabled me to reflect upon many of my values and beliefs about nursing. It made me even more passionate about nursing's place beside the patient and even more in awe of those who demonstrated expertise in their professional craft, but probably would not have dared to call themselves an expert. This has resulted in the generation of a philosophy of caring, built on personal experience, an assimilation of research evidence and review of the literature on the subject.

The third conceptual building block was to spend time in critical care practice: first, to see if this personal philosophy had any currency in contemporary critical care practice; and secondly to capture the issues and concerns of critical care practitioners, notably around how to facilitate their colleagues and find strategies to keep themselves motivated and strategic in their career trajectories. In the Autumn of 2004 I returned to ITU to undertake clinical practice as a health care assistant. Once again, this significant learning transition helped me to reflect, consider and contemplate my values and beliefs. Although a short time in practice, this was a powerful learning experience and one that fundamentally shaped the construction of this book.

The book uses vignettes from fieldwork, teaching experience and the experience of being a patient to illustrate key theoretical points. They are used to inform reflective comparison with the contemporary literature on the subject, to challenge, explore and offer an alternative mode of looking at the issue. These have been stylistically separated and flagged in the text to help the reader ascertain the source of each illustration. It is hoped that this approach will assist those engaged in reflective writing to foster their own unique style. Importantly the vignettes are there to illustrate the theory I am proposing: that iteration between critical reflection on experience, the literature and research findings can trigger new insights into familiar problems or serve to strengthen the knowledge, values and beliefs that underpin our care. Names in the vignettes have been changed to protect people's anonymity.

I hope that the perspectives set out in this text, which are sometimes controversial, add to the debates about professional critical care practice. My hope is that these will stimulate practitioners to reflect on and consider how they can enhance their practice and strive towards the goal of expertise in critical care nursing.

Julie Scholes

Acknowledgements

This book is built upon research findings arising from field work and analysis undertaken by myself and colleagues. Findings from these studies have been selected to theoretically examine career transitions in critical care nursing. The views expressed in this book are those of the author and may not necessarily be shared by former colleagues or the commissioners of the research. Every effort has been made to ensure that there are no errors in the book, but, if there are any, they are entirely attributable to me.

Two colleagues have contributed to this book: John Albarran, co-editor on BACCN's journal *Nursing in Critical Care*, and Professor Caroline Williams, a former research student. When one meets inspirational nurse leaders and educators who share a passion for excellence in nursing and are driven to see the possibilities of critical care nursing being realised, it serves to energise, strengthen and motivate. Caroline and John are two such people who have tirelessly sought to enable others to realise their potential as critical care nurses. They have generously contributed to this book, offering alternative perspectives that serve to broaden and strengthen the analysis in the book.

The list of colleagues with whom I have worked is extensive but the following should be mentioned who have been involved in research that has been included in this book:

Professor Ruth Endacott, Dr Marnie Freeman, Professor Morag Gray, Dr Gerri Matthews Smith, Dilys Robinson, Bernadette Wallis, Professor Carolyn Miller, Matthew Moore, Melanie Smith, Annie Chellel, Professor Christine Webb, Professor Melanie Jasper, Professor Barbara Vaughan, and the research team on the ENRiP study notably Professor Sue Read and Abigail Masterson. Each one of these inspirational researchers, educators and leaders has shaped my thinking and broadened my perspectives and offered friendship, humour and motivation to keep pursuing the elusive goal of discovering how to enable others to achieve expertise in nursing.

In addition, there are a network of colleagues with whom I link at conferences, who have inspired, critiqued and added to the body of knowledge through their own research and practice developments. Importantly, there are all the students who I have had the privilege of teaching, and research participants who have shared their experiences with me: too many to name, but you know who you are. This book is both for and about you. I hope it provides you with a toolkit to enable you to achieve your potential and facilitate those you mentor to do the same. It is hoped this book provides you with the confidence to take up your rightful and privileged position beside the patient and that the reworking of your issues into the various chapters of this book does justice to your commitment, motivation and energy.

Finally there are colleagues who have specifically assisted with the development of this manuscript: to Beth Knight, Commissioning Editor, and Katharine Taylor, Editorial Assistant in the Professional Department at Blackwells, for their patience and help in the development of this manuscript.

Cathy McGuiness, Practice Educator for adult critical care, Brighton and Sussex University Hospitals Trust, for providing some examples of recognising weaknesses in students' and colleagues' performance. Jim Valentine, clinical manager for adult critical care, Brighton and Sussex University Hospitals Trust, for facilitating my return to practice and Jane Butler, Acting Head of Nursing, Brighton and Sussex University Hospitals Trust, for allowing this to happen.

Dr Alec Grant, Caroline Leach and Annie Chellel for their invaluable feedback on early drafts of the chapters and providing critical support.

I would like to acknowledge the support of the ENB in commissioning the research underlying the report *Evaluation of the effectiveness of educational preparation for critical care nursing* (Scholes and Endacott, 2002) and the subsequent support of the NUC following its take over of the ENB in 2002.

Author profiles

Professor Julie Scholes *DPhil, MSc (Nursing), DipN, DANS, RN*
Professor of Nursing, Centre for Nursing and Midwifery Research, University of Brighton

Julie's clinical background is in critical care nursing. Since 1987 she has been in nurse education and since 1993 her primary role has been in research. She is particularly interested in practice developments that arise from the implementation of research findings. Her research activities link back to the way in which education impacts upon the development of practice, and she prides herself on the fact that much of her research is conducted in practice settings.

She has been involved in a number of research projects. Recently these include: the evaluation of the new model of pre-registration provision, the *Making a Difference* Curriculum (commissioned by the Department of Health); an evaluation and generation of core competencies for critical care nursing (commissioned by the ENB); an evaluation of the use of portfolios to demonstrate clinical competence (commissioned by the ENB); and an evaluation of critical care Outreach services (with Kent Critical Care Network). Current research includes: an evaluation of how educational preparation enables the non-medical workforce to undertake new ways of working: an action research project examining the transformation of culture to achieve greater time for scholarship and research; developments in the link lecturer role; and the impact of teacher exchange on educationalists and students. She is now working with a number of colleagues facilitating their research and building research links with the local Trusts. She is Co-editor of *Nursing in Critical Care*

John W. Albarran *Msc Advanced Nursing Practice, BSc (Hons), PG DipEd, DipN (Lon), RN, NFESC*
Principal Lecturer in Critical Care, University of the West of England, Bristol

John Albarran is a registered nurse and academic with over 20 years' critical care nursing experience based at the Faculty of Health and Social Care at the University of the West of England, Bristol, United Kingdom.

John has been an active national board member of the British Association of Critical Care Nurses for 14 years and has played a strategic role in the development and progress of the Association. Together with Professor Julie Scholes, John co-edits the journal *Nursing in Critical Care* on behalf of the Association. Last year John was elected to the executive committee of the European Federation of Critical Care Nursing Associations. He is also a former member of the World Federation of Critical Care Nurses (2000–05). Other professional roles include participating as chair or member of scientific committees of national and international conferences.

John's research and publication interests are broad and diverse and revolve around: role developments of critical care, advanced practice, acute cardiac symptoms and differential diagnosis, resuscitation, and nutrition of ICU patients. He has co-authored one text on principles of intensive care nursing, and three chapters relating to critical care issues and advanced nursing practice. His most recent text with Pam Moule, *Practical Resuscitation: Recognition and Response*, was published last year by Blackwell Publications. John has also presented papers at major international conferences.

Professor Caroline Williams *PhD, BSc (Hons), RGN, DPSN, PGCert (Res) Commander in Queen Alexandra's Royal Naval Nursing Service (QARNNS), Head of School for the Defence School of Health Care Studies, Royal Centre for Defence Medicine and University of Central England, Birmingham*

Caroline qualified as a registered nurse in Dundee, Scotland and completed her critical care nursing course in Edinburgh before joining the Royal Navy in 1989. Following tours of duty in the UK and Gibraltar, Caroline moved into nurse education, whilst retaining her passion for critical care. Experiencing the challenges across both pre- and post-registration education delivery, she was appointed as Nurse Education Advisor for the Royal Navy in 1999, and was promoted to Commander and Head of the Defence School of Health Care Studies in 2004. In July 2003, Caroline became the first defence nurse to gain a PhD, and in 2005 was awarded her Professorship by the University of Central England in recognition of her leadership and ongoing contribution to the development of health care education within the Defence Medical Services.

With clinical roots firmly in adult intensive care, Caroline's research and publication interests are focused around the psychological care of patients in ICU. This led to her doctoral study which sought to unearth the subtle and often hidden aspects of nurse–patient interaction in the intensive care setting. This study highlighted the unique role that the nurse, through effective communication, can play in helping patients to adapt to the ICU environment, enhancing patients' experiences of care, and mediating many of the factors that may serve to promote or hinder their adaptation and recovery.

Part 1
Theoretical pillars and political context of developing expertise in critical care

Chapter 1
Expertise in critical care

Introduction

Critical care practice is challenging. It requires continuous thoughtful and intelligent engagement with patients and their relatives and with colleagues. To do this effectively the practitioner requires high levels of energy, emotional resilience and a broad knowledge to respond to the dynamic context of practice and rapidly changing clinical situations (Benner *et al.*, 1999). Performance has to be skilful and empathic to be constructed as competent (Scholes and Endacott, 2002). There is little margin for error but huge potential to make a significant difference and this can be evidenced in the smallest gesture, thought, word or deed, as much as in bold and creative interventions. Much of critical care involves the application of leading edge health care technologies, medicines and treatment modalities, but such interventions only increase the need for enhanced, empathic, fundamental care. Experts bring together all these elements and display them through professional artistry and sound clinical judgement (Titchen and Higgs, 2001).

This chapter sets out to identify what expertise is and how others might be facilitated to realise it. Theoretical descriptors distilled from the literature are presented to illustrate how expertise can be recognised. As rapid clinical decision making is crucial in expert critical care practice, a brief review of the factors involved is presented to gain a purchase on how this might be taught to, or researched by, others. Then a model of learning transition theory is introduced. The final section turns to how these core concepts have given the book its structure, and provides an overview of each chapter to enable the reader to zero in on areas that have most relevance to their current activity, learning or facilitation cycle to help them on their personal journey towards expertise.

First, my task is to clarify my own values and beliefs about the nature of expertise. The intention is to offer transparency so the reader can establish how the issues debated have been influenced by my own perceptual filter. They are that:

(1) Expertise is not the sole province of clinicians in senior positions at the pinnacle of their profession. Elements of expertise can be achieved at various stages on the journey through one's clinical career. Senior colleagues

might have a broader repertoire of expert performance than that of more junior colleagues who demonstrate expertise in very specific activities.

(2)   Expertise is context specific, the context being care of the critically ill, wherever they, the patients, are located.

(3)   Expertise is evident when the practitioner is able to respond to complex situations with ease, precision and fluidity, which inspire confidence in others. It is demonstrated by individuals who have mastery of both applied scientific and craft knowledge and who demonstrate mastery of their practice environment and the technology to support the critically ill patient.

(4)   The changing dynamic of practice knowledge and the aspiration to develop and progress clinical practice to better fit the needs of patients and their relatives drive experts to develop more expertise. Expertise by its very nature is therefore both transitory and sometimes elusive.

(5)   Expertise is not a plateau on to which one can climb, then sit back and relax to enjoy the view. It is a constantly evolving process and the aspiration to achieve it inspires and energises. Every critical care practitioner should continuously strive to develop and demonstrate expertise within their sphere of practice, and build their repertoire of skills and knowledge in line with the latest technological advances. Senior clinicians, by their nature, are at the leading edge of developing critical care practice, but innovative practice will require consolidation before it can be construed as expert practice.

(6)   Expertise improves patients' and their relatives' experience of the critical care service and this outcome makes the pursuit of expertise an enormously rewarding journey for the practitioner.

(7)   To be expert in all aspects of one's role could be perceived as an ideal state. Most practitioners will demonstrate aspects of expertise in certain areas of their practice whilst aspiring to expertise in other components of their role. Like a graphic equaliser, these peak at different moments in time but require energy and investment to keep them towards the top end of their potential. Assessment of current performance is key to initiate progression in weaker areas and to sustain areas of high level performance. This feedback loop motivates the practitioner to continue in their quest to attain expert practice.

(8)   Outward objective markers are not necessarily conterminous with expertise. Some roles require there to be evidence of clinical, educational, leadership or research expertise as a standard for the appointment or conferment of a title (e.g. consultant nurse), but most would expect this to develop further with the experience of being in the post. One might assume some degree of expertise in a subject because an individual has a range of qualifications. However, when one gets down to the core of what makes a critical care nurse an expert, neither a title nor a qualification necessarily confirms this is the case: these simply map the journey taken in the pursuit of expertise and the context in which they practise.

(9)   Expertise is recognisable to patients and their relatives, and to students and colleagues. It is a way of being with patients and their relatives that creates therapeutic presence.

(10)   Expert critical care nursing is an art form, comforting to experience, moving to watch, inspirational to encounter.

What is expertise? A review of the literature

Expertise is a relative condition that confers status and confirms that one individual has attributes, skills or knowledge at a higher level than another (Jasper, 1994). Therefore, at whatever stage in their clinical career, the individual may possess elements of expertise relative to others. The knowledge, skills and abilities of an 'expert' are acquired throughout the clinical career from practice learning encounters supplemented by academic studies. They are refined and honed by clinical experience. They can be facilitated by others who enable the transitioner to realise their potential through reflective engagement and review.

Others may look at an expert and give them the label, whilst the individual upon whom this compliment has been bestowed shyly rejects such a notion. Indeed, using the principle that the more we know the more we realise that we don't know, the self-proclaimed state of expertise could never be achieved. Experience seems a far more comfortable construct to claim for oneself.

Conway (1996) argues that there are four types of expertise. These are influenced by the organisational setting in which the individual works, their speciality, and the worldview of the practitioner. She identified that each typology of expertise uses different forms of knowledge in different ways. First, there is the category of 'technologists' (who use a wide range of knowledge including anticipatory, diagnostic and technical knowhow and monitoring). Secondly, there are the 'traditionalists' (who mainly use medical knowledge; ironically, within the current health care workforce, this typology is most likely to refer to practitioners in a variety of new roles where medical substitution is prevalent). Thirdly, there are 'specialists' (who use knowledge of assessment, diagnosis and quality of life and often assume the role of clinical nurse specialists). Finally, there are the 'humanistic existentialists' (considered to practise from a holistic practice perspective and who use a range of theoretical knowledge and experiential wisdom underpinned by teaching from nursing and social science (Conway, 1996)). In the decade that has passed since Conway's original research, role developments have been rapid, radical and extensive. It is now more likely that nurses have to demonstrate expertise in more than one domain, and like a chameleon take on the guise that is necessary, especially when working to a broad range of competencies or assuming multiple sub-roles (such as a consultant nurse). Within the speciality of critical care, it would be an expectation for consultant nurses to demonstrate technical expertise within an holistic model of care. This would be a relative position to a junior colleague who might well be a 'technical expert' without necessarily having the breadth and depth of knowledge and experiential wisdom to inform clinical decisions beyond a very focused sphere of practice.

We can aspire to excellence in nursing (which hinges upon notions of caring, empathy and presencing) at any stage in our career or within our sphere of practice. However, writers do link experiential wisdom and excellence with expertise (e.g. Benner *et al.*, 1996; Titchen and Higgs, 2001). To achieve such a state requires active teaching and learning (Benner *et al.*, 1996) or critical companionship[1] (Titchen, 2001). Furthermore, to sustain expertise, one needs to nourish it with new knowledge and experience and hydrate it with critical scrutiny and constructive, reflective analysis to keep the condition evolving and growing. This can be achieved by building theory from practice for practice, by facilitating experiential learning in self and others, and by critical evaluation of one's own practice from the perspective of the client (Titchen, 2001). Thus we turn full circle to the idea that expertise is a journey rather than a destination, and that critical reflection is the vehicle in which that journey is made, and the acquisition of new theoretical and experiential knowledge the energy to fuel the vehicle.

To adopt such an approach is proactive and intentional. Dreyfus and Dreyfus (1986) argue that most expert performance is on-going and non-reflective unless confronted with an unusual or critical situation. Even in these situations, the expert tends to reflect upon their intuitive decision making rather than their problem solving *per se* (Dreyfus and Dreyfus, 1986). This is what enables there to be fluidity, salience and artistry in their performance, and that is what distinguishes their practice from that of others. Therefore, to make everyday practice of the expert unusual, it needs to be examined through a critically reflective research, teaching or leadership lens. This is not to impede the expert, but to ensure that they review what they do and seek to enhance their performance and the practice of their colleagues. Sharing of expertise is critical for succession planning, but herein lies the challenge for the 'expert': they know what they do but making explicit to others how they do it is a problem when it is so embodied in their personal knowing.

In part what an expert has is something of the mystical or an indefinable quality that is revered by others (Paterson and Zderad, 1976). They have the ability to capture the essence of a complex scenario and zero in on the important issues and act appropriately without the use of standardised diagnostic principles (Benner and Tanner, 1987; Jasper, 1994). Knowledge, experience and skill are a fluid interplay that iterates between past and new experience and manifests as skilled artistry or craft knowledge (Titchen and Higgs, 2001),

---

[1] Critical companionship has three defining characteristics: skilled companionship (or being patient centred), being self-reflective and self-evaluative, and being able to create and critically review professional craft knowledge. Some methods to enhance these skills have been outlined in the final sections of Chapters 6 and 7.

'knowhow' (Gatley, 1992) or 'tacit knowledge' (Polanyi, 1967). It is often hard for the expert to explicitly set out their decision-making process; although there is such a process, it is often self-devised strategies rather than general rules or operational strategies that govern what they know and do (Benner,1984) or their 'performance [is] without conscious awareness of the knowledge being used' (Woolery, 1990).

Some, notably Benner, link 'unconscious performance' with intuition. Eraut (1994) challenges the assumption that intuition informs the expert's decision making. Rather, the expert possesses the capacity to deliberate and analyse, under conditions where rapid interpretation of data and decision making are required to inform skilled actions. Rarely is theory taken off the shelf and used in practice without its first being personalised and integrated into the conceptual frameworks of the practitioner (Eraut, 1994: 157), and this process of synthesis and application makes the decision making seem mystical, intuitive or inaccessible to anyone other than that 'expert'. But such assumptions take no account of the proportion of the expert professional's practice that is said to be 'intuitive'. Is it that exceptionally wise and salient decisions are given disproportionate weighting by an awed collegiate audience? To what extent do reputation and regard blind us to the possibility of 'expert fallibility' (Eraut, 1994:128), or fail to tell us where this type of 'intuitive' decision making is, in fact, wrong? Most importantly, we need to develop a deeper understanding of how we can enable others to master the talents, knowledge and skill to achieve this type of decision making and reduce the rate of error. To do this we need critical, purposive self-evaluation and an audit of the outcomes of the clinical interventions made by the expert nurse, but also more research into how those clinical judgements were reached. But once again this raises a number of challenges, not least of which are:

- breaking down the anatomy of the 'expert's' clinical decision making; and
- isolating the variable of the 'expert's' subsequent intervention.

Role modelling clinical decision making

Much of the research into clinical decision making has focused on medical staff. In determining diagnosis, medics have been identified as focusing on a working hypothesis which narrows the field of reasoning around the chief complaint or data obtained in the first minutes of interaction with the patient. Thus they can work back through diagnostic criteria to alight upon the range of investigations that are required to confirm or refute their diagnostic hypothesis (Elstein and Bordage, 1979). However, to do this relies heavily upon memory to draw out the most salient hypothesis (Eraut, 1994). For the majority, experience is essential to keep one's memory banks attuned, updated and linked to the most contemporary investigations. This is the reason why expertise is so often linked with the currency of experience in a specialist area.

Secondly, although there is a risk of error, the scope of investigations that can be ordered can, from past experience, be determined to yield the most reliable results or broadest opportunity to further locate a more refined working hypothesis (limited only by financial constraints). We can reflect upon this in critical care medicine, where the intensivist is ordering investigations to confirm their initial or subjective data with the 'scientific proof' of results. Care bundles, protocols and guidelines are methods for standardising investigations and procedures and also serve to reduce the risk of relying solely on the practitioner's memory. However, they require an accurate diagnostic hypothesis in the first instance. The 'hunting in herds' or medical ward round is often seen as a complex interplay of questions and answers to help the intensivist eliminate a range of hypothetical diagnoses by bouncing their ideas or articulating their thinking and seeking confirmation from the rest of the team that they are on the right track. To what extent could a nursing ward round led by a clinical expert hone in on clinical nursing decisions on the critical care unit, and refine and make explicit their clinical decision making? The potential and power of this type of learning and dissemination of expertise have never been fully realised. Why should this be the case?

Little has been invested in examining the decision-making processes of the expert nurse. Benner's work does not provide an anatomical dissection of the way knowledge is processed, filtered and synthesised to form a diagnosis. Rather, it focuses on clinical inquiry, clinical grasp, clinical forethought and experiential learning and how these impact upon expert performance in practice (Lynaugh, 1999). Benner and her colleagues (1999) argue that through the use of expert nurses' narrative we can understand how they formulate judgements that are based upon knowing the patient over a period of time and judging any change in their condition by looking for trends in their presentation and comparing these with experience of other illness trajectories. Situated clinical decision making is essential for learning this professional skill and they caution that:

> 'the matching of patient findings against a predefined template or the application of artificial intelligence can provide decision support, but can never replace the engaged clinical and ethical reasoning of the clinician whose judgement is shaped by the context of the situation.' (Benner et al., 1999: xi).

They argue that, through the sharing of narrative or dialogue, others may come to understand this embodied knowledge.[2] What is critical is to get this articulated and shared on a regular basis. The (re)introduction of the nursing ward round, led by a critical care nurse who has expertise in clinical nursing

---

[2] This has significance for the methodological approach to the examination of experts' clinical decision making, i.e. the importance for it to be in the real world of clinical practice to capture the situational, temporal and dynamic complexity of formulating advanced clinical judgements. Simulated environments and/or scenarios can only serve to make synthetic or formulaic responses which would belie the true complexity of experts' decision-making processes.

judgements, would provide the forum for specific coaching in clinical decision making that is grounded in a model of compassionate, moral and ethical practice. To enable this to really be effective, such rounds would have to take place in a climate of mutual respect. Alternatively, such narratives could be shared in group clinical supervision sessions (see Chapter 6). However, although this may seem initially more comfortable, it removes the clinical decision-making process away from the patient and the clinical setting (and thereby reduces the possibility of temporal and situational assessment).

Wise ethical and clinical judgements are reached by situational analysis, and are steeped in the relationship the nurse has with the patient. To fully understand all the complexity of decision making, we need far greater insight into the processes involved, but also need to celebrate such expertise and to see it shared in more open and constructively challenging clinical situations. Put simply, we need to see more of our clinical nursing experts making their decisions before a group of nurses (and hopefully, a researcher). But this is not a task isolated to clinical leaders. Every individual with expertise relative to a colleague needs to be part of the project to encourage transitions towards expertise. To do this we need to habitually narrate what we do to others and question their *understanding* of the experience.

This approach has become somewhat out of vogue since the introduction of reflective practice whereby the individual is encouraged to distil their own knowledge and understanding of a situation or experience through reflective writing or in dialogue with another. Further, the postmodernist rejection of professional expertise in favour of public access to knowledge has further diminished the enthusiasm to share relative understanding with others. Narration requires the articulation of applied knowledge in the real time of action rather than assuming a learner has acquired an understanding of the situation by being there and checking this out through *post hoc* accounts of the experience. Narration of action illuminates what there is to be learnt and can help to identify important elements of craft knowledge and professional artistry that may not be immediately obvious to someone with less experience. This is not to suggest that narration and questioning should be adopted in favour of reflection, rather that both approaches complement one another, reinforce learning and are critical to the project of facilitating transitions to expertise. This helps the learner identify what there is to be learnt, and for the narrator this helps them to speak of what they already know and identify what more they need to know to enhance or refresh their relative expertise.

Expert clinical leaders set the tone and model a style of practice that others might seek to emulate (Spinosa *et al.*, 1997). They generate environments in which individuals are enabled to take personal risks and offer possibilities to learn new ways of practising that empower that individual but also enhance patient care. Clinical experts act as catalysts who stimulate the possibility of change in practice for the individual and the clinical community (RCN Institute, 2002). They have to act with courage and fortitude (Benner *et al.*, 1999) and sometimes function as mavericks to bring about radical change within potentially stagnant organisations (RCN Institute, 2002). Reaching out to enable individuals to make change and then being rewarded by watching the nurse transition into the next stage of their personal journey towards expertise becomes a dynamic evolving force that sustains the effort. At the same time, they need to see when an individual is functioning outside their sphere of competence and take remedial action to either rectify that or reframe the range of responsibilities that the individual is expected to fulfil. They also need to ensure that organisational expediency does not result in the delegation of caring responsibilities to non-professional practitioners that place the patient at risk (Benner *et al.*, 1999).

The chapter now goes on to present a model of role transition and how relative experts can facilitate their colleagues to achieve their potential.

The journey to expertise: the learning transitions model

Critical in the developmental journey towards expertise is how various learning experiences affect the individual. This book's focus is on learning transitions and how they affect professional development.

Have you ever wondered why some people might encounter a learning opportunity (e.g. a course, study day, collegiate supervision or grade change) and seem apparently untouched by the experience, whereas, for others, this same learning opportunity results in significant professional and personal change? This is because of the degree of turbulence new learning generates in existing understanding. Put simply, when an individual encounters new information or an experience that **confirms** their beliefs and values (be they professional or personal), and that expands their repertoire of abilities and understanding, there is *developmental* change. However, if an individual is exposed to an alternative perspective that challenges past constructs or understanding, and this new perspective **contradicts** past assumptions or values, this will have a significant impact on the individual and will trigger the *transformation* of knowledge and practice.

In some instances the cascade of change can be quite radical, resulting in altered behaviour not only in the workplace but also in personal and social life. Conversely, life event transitions can either enhance or detract from the individual's professional performance. The learning that takes place from these experiences and how they inform professional performance can be harnessed by facilitated reflective insight, assessment, appraisal or review. However, some individuals can **actively resist** or **defend against** the possibility of any change because of the potential cascade dynamic that can follow. This is evident among individuals who are emotionally or socially vulnerable and fear any shift in the status quo. However, if they have sufficient support (environmental, emotional, educational and social), these individuals can have the most profound transformative transitions. But a facilitator should be cautious. It may be necessary for foundational work to build self-esteem and

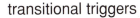

transitional triggers

contradictory experiential learning

professional development

qualification change

grade change

awareness: compensatory confirming

developmental: professional maturation

transformative: reflective redefining

transitional models

Fig. 1.1 Experiential triggers and a taxonomy of professional transitions (Scholes, 1995).

confidence before an individual feels able to face *any* change (Fennell, 1999). In certain cases, trained therapists rather than colleagues or educationalists should undertake this.

Not all transitions are linear and in an upward trajectory. But as a rule of thumb, the greater the disturbance the more profound the transitional experience, especially where this is closely tied to the individual's identity. Figure 1.1 sets out different types of transition and the key characteristic which differentiates the experience for the transitioner.

Although some transitions will be triggered by formal educational experiences, by far the majority occur through learning from experiences in practice. The following conditions (personal and external) are required to effectively transform knowledge and practice and thereby stimulate transitions towards expertise in the practice setting (see Fig. 1.2).

Tolerating contradiction is key to experiential learning and this can be triggered by critical, evaluative reflection to ultimately achieve the transformation of knowledge and practice. However, this requires the practitioner to be open to revisit past assumptions in the light of new knowledge and experiences, and that requires an environment that is built on trust, support and facilitation and stimulates a culture of high challenge and high support (Manley, 2000).

The current trend to avoid repetition in formal educational provision (Scholes and Chellel, 1999) can result in the spiral or iterative cycles of reflecting and revisiting, and deepening understanding, becoming less likely in the academic setting as the student is encouraged to move on to study new topics. However, in practice, health care professionals are constantly exposed to similar clinical incidents and an array of alternative strategies for their management, which can trigger the transformation of knowledge and practice. If the individual is open and willing to review this, or when such encounters are accompanied

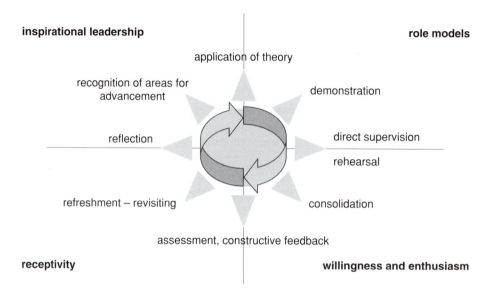

Fig. 1.2 Conditions to effect learning from practice.

by facilitated reflection by an inspirational teacher or expert role model, it strengthens the potential learning power of the experience. However, the expert needs to stand back and seek evaluation from their colleague about what has helped them to develop their practice and thinking so they might equip themselves with a repertoire of helping strategies that are effective to others (Benner *et al.*, 1999). When such experiences are repeated and contradiction becomes an expectation of their experiential learning, the knowledge and skills become embodied by the nurse, who is well on their way to achieving expertise and excellence in critical care nursing.

The context in which the practitioner works has a powerful impact on learning how to learn or indeed on creating an environment which embraces transformative learning as an integral component of its culture (Manley, 2000). But the individual has to expose themselves to these learning opportunities: one does not go without the other. If a practitioner remains closed off to the possibility of learning through contradiction, they cannot ultimately achieve transformed understanding. The most powerful effect is often obtained where the familiar is rendered strange by seeing practice from another perspective.

The antithesis to this is routinised practice delivered by burnt-out, care-less practitioners struggling against the demands of each day. This rut is a self-fulfilling downward spiral as each day seems to be more demanding and a fight against negativity. Therefore, critical to turning this position into a positive experience is a willingness and enthusiasm to see things from a different perspective: for example, to experience the contradiction that they *can* positively impact upon practice and patient care. The guidance and facilitation of an enthusiastic colleague are important in enabling the individual to find their way back out on to the positive spiral towards achieving transformative learning and ultimately expertise.

Chapter overview

The book has been divided into three key sections. The first section sets out the theoretical pillars and political context of developing expertise in critical care. The second section turns to address how role transition theory can be used to facilitate self and others on their journey towards expertise. The final section sets out the new ways of working that affect critical care provision within the contemporary NHS. The material in this book has been collated to enable the reader to focus on certain aspects that meet their needs at any given time. Therefore, some topics are referred to in more than one chapter, especially where this is critical to the completeness of that chapter. To enable readers to select the most appropriate chapters to meet their needs, they are guided to the index but also the chapter summary below.

In Chapter 2, I set out a personal philosophy of caring and argue that, when realised, such performance can be viewed as clinical excellence in nursing. The chapter concludes with an examination of the factors that can inhibit the achievement of excellence in care. It seeks to stimulate those wishing to reflect on their own philosophy of caring, especially if their personal values and beliefs have been challenged by events or circumstances.

In Chapter 3, Caroline Williams has provided a comprehensive and persuasive account of the contextual dynamics that challenge critical care nurses in transition towards expertise. She draws together a complex array of policy directives and agendas to clearly demarcate the issues, and provides the foundation on which the remaining arguments of the book are located. This chapter is expected to be of particular interest to people starting out in their critical care career or students studying the political dynamics of service provision.

The theoretical model for examining the change process that individuals encounter when they progress through their career is role transition. This has been used to make sense of experiences, some of which may be incredibly painful and others seemingly insignificant, that we encounter as we transition through our career, all building up to tell the story of how we strive to achieve expertise in critical care nursing. Importantly, the examination of our own personal role transitions can help us to meaningfully facilitate others with their learning transitions. Chapter 4 provides an examination and analysis of role, career and learning transition theory, drawing upon experiential vignettes and fieldwork observations to illustrate the issues as applied to the critical care context.

From here the book moves on to describe ways of learning and support to facilitate learning transitions towards expertise throughout the clinical career. In Chapter 5 formal educational strategies are addressed which include the provision of pre- and post-registration education pathways and are critically examined to analyse how they enable the acquisition of knowledge and competence for critical care practice. This section is written for practitioners who are struggling to enable a reluctant learner to acquire the necessary critical care skills and knowledge, and provides a resource of different options to effect learning.

Chapter 6 addresses different strategies that can be deployed within the workbase to facilitate practitioner development. This includes facilitating horizontal learning transitions as well as upward career development. This chapter is expected to be of interest to anyone who either facilitates their colleagues or is about to embark on a new role within the critical care arena.

Chapter 7 goes on to examine the role of assessment and how this can be used as a learning and developmental strategy. Issues related to the assessment of students on formal programmes, as well as evaluation of colleagues' clinical performance, are reviewed. This section is expected to be of interest to students who are undertaking programmes of study that enhance their role as mentors. The final section of this chapter may be of use to individuals strategically planning their career path as it explores different self-assessment strategies that they can adopt to help them to constantly iterate through the action, evaluation and practice development cycles critical for the pursuit, sustenance and consolidation of expertise.

Chapter 8 addresses how the modernisation agenda of workforce redesign has been structured and how competency frameworks have been used to re-engineer roles and redefine cross-boundary working at various rungs of the clinical career ladder. It offers a critical analysis of competencies and of how they enable practitioner development. The example of the critical care practitioner is used to illustrate these main themes, and the chapter concludes with an analysis of the factors which might inhibit the proliferation of such roles. This chapter is likely to be of interest to those who are either engaged in competency development for their staff or involved in enabling new workers to work differently to meet staff resource deficits, or simply to enhance practitioners' understanding of the dynamic context of change they experience in their everyday work.

In Chapter 9, John Albarran has provided a critical review of the way new roles have developed, notably in the field of coronary care. He challenges the assumption that some of these new roles exemplify nursing expertise or indeed advanced practice. He starts by mapping different types of nurse-led roles and knowledge in use on a continuum from the substitution of medical tasks through to autonomous practice. He then firmly asserts that protocolised, substitution roles fall outwith any notion of nursing expertise because there is no room for autonomy, diagnosis, referral or decision making. Practitioners undertaking new roles in critical care practice will find John Albarran's critical review of the issues inherent to the inception and expansion of these roles an invaluable resource to enable them to guard against some of the risks and accentuate the positive aspects of new role development.

Chapter 10 examines some of the challenges which face our leaders and expert practitioners in the future, and explores the new range of knowledge and skills they will have to acquire to meet these new demands and assert their rightful place beside the patient. It concludes with a survival kit to help to foster, nurture and sustain the energy and dynamism required of those on their journey towards expertise.

References

Benner P (1984) *From Novice to Expert: Excellence and Power in Clinical Nursing.* Menlo Park, California: Addison-Wesley.

Benner P and Tanner C (1987) Clinical judgement: how expert nurses use intuition. *American Journal of Nursing* **87**: 23–31.

Benner P, Tanner C and Chesla C (1996) *Expertise in Nursing Practice Caring, Clinical Judgement and Ethics.* New York: Springer Publishing.

Benner P, Hooper-Kyriakidis P and Stannard D (1999) *Clinical Wisdom and Interventions in Critical care: A Thinking-in-Action Approach.* Philadelphia: WB Saunders.

Conway J (1996) *Nursing Expertise and Advanced Practice.* Salisbury Quay Books: Mark Allen Publishing.

Dreyfus H and Dreyfus S (1986) *Mind over Machine: the Power of Human Intuition and Expertise in the Era of the Computer.* Oxford: Basil Blackwell.

Elstein AS and Bordage G (1979) Psychology of clinical reasoning. In Stone G, Cohen F and Adler NE (eds). *Health Psychology: A Handbook.* San Francisco: Jossey Bass.

Eraut M (1994) *Developing Professional Knowledge and Competence.* London: Falmer Press.

Fennell M (1999) *Overcoming Low Self-esteem: A Self-help Guide Using Cognitive Behavioural Techniques.* London: Robinson.

Gatley E (1992) From novice to expert: the use of intuitive knowledge as a basis for district nurse education. *Nurse Education Today* **12**: 81–87.

Jasper M (1994) Expert: a discussion on the implications of the concept as used in nursing. *Journal of Advanced Nursing* **20**: 769–776.

Lynaugh J (1999) Foreword 1. In: Benner, P, Hooper-Kyriakidis P and Stannard, D (eds). *Clinical Wisdom and Interventions in Critical Care: A Thinking-in-Action Approach.* Philadelphia: WB Saunders.

Manley K (2000) Organisational culture and consultant nurse outcomes: Part 1 – Organisational culture. *Nursing in Critical Care* **5**(4): 179–184.

Paterson J and Zderad L (1976) *Humanistic Nursing.* New York: John Wiley and Sons.

Polanyi M (1967) *The Tacit Dimension.* London: Routledge.

Royal College of Nursing Institute (RCN Institute) (2002) *Expertise in Practice Project: Exploring Expertise.* London: RCN.

Scholes J (1995) An exploration of role transition in students converting from Enrolled Nurse (General) to Registered General Nurse (Unpublished DPhil, Sussex University).

Scholes J and Chellel A (1999) Pulled in all directions: Tutors' accounts of managing critical care courses. *Nursing in Critical Care* **4**(1): 34–39.

Scholes J and Endacott R (2002) *Evaluation of the Effectiveness of Educational Preparation for Critical Care Nursing.* London: ENB, available from www.nmc-uk.org.

Spinosa C, Flores F and Dreyfus H (1997) *Disclosing New Worlds: Entrepreneurship, Democratic Action, and the Cultivation of Solidarity.* Cambridge, MA: MIT.

Titchen A (2001) Critical companionship: a conceptual framework for developing expertise. In Higgs J and Tichen A (eds). *Practice Knowledge and Expertise in the Health Professions.* Oxford: Butterworth Heinemann.

Titchen A and Higgs J (2001) A dynamic framework for the enhancement of health professional practice in an uncertain world: the practice–knowledge interface. In Higgs J and Titchen A (eds). *Practice Knowledge and Expertise in the Health Professions.* Oxford: Butterworth Heinemann.

Woolery L (1990) Expert nurses and expert systems. *Computers in Nursing* **8**: 23–27.

Chapter 2
Critical to care: towards a model of caring excellence

*'Nurses provide care for people in the midst of health, pain, loss, fear, disfigurement, death, grieving, challenge, growth, birth and transition on an intimate and front line basis. Expert nurses call this **the privileged place of nursing**.'* (Benner and Wrubel, 1989: xi).

Introduction

This chapter sets out a model of caring excellence that is an aspirational standard of practice for all critical care nurses and therefore can be seen as core to any notion of expertise in nursing practice. Through the use of reflective vignettes it illuminates examples of practice and draws upon the literature to debate what should be considered the core values of nursing and how they might be realised in our everyday interaction with the patient. Examples of indifferent practice are presented to help distinguish that which is excellent. These examples specifically focus upon the minutiae of an interaction that make up the art of nursing, and upon how, when this art fuses with scientific knowhow and technical expertise, this transforms to the status of excellent care.

The chapter then goes on to debate some of the factors identified from research that might impede the art of nursing from being realised. From this basis the rest of the book builds to identify ways to facilitate learning transitions that trigger the potential for transformation to excellent carer in various stages of career progression.

The dose of nursing

Watching an excellent nurse, one can see something in her practice that makes you want to capture it and spread it to others. There is a natural elegance in the interactions with patients, an harmonious interplay that sets the patient and the relatives at their ease, comfortable in the knowledge that they are in safe hands. The presence of such a nurse has of itself a therapeutic quality and this has been termed by Norris (2000) the 'dose of nursing'. Conversely, the absence of excellence is equally observable and recently much lamented (e.g. Magnet, 2003). Magnet's critique of nursing followed a period of two weeks in hospital. Suffering from a complex autoimmune disease, she had experienced a number of hospitalisations which she felt positioned her as an 'expert on hospitals' (ibid.). Magnet complained that the nurses she encountered seemed neither technically competent nor kind and caring. Her perspective on the decline of modern nursing was reinforced in a report produced by Sergent of the Centre for Policy Studies. Following an 11-month study of the NHS, Sergent (2003) concluded that there was a lack of concern about the quality of care in the NHS. Similarly, the evaluation of the 'new' nursing curriculum concluded that, although pockets of excellence were evident, it was far more common to hear about, or see, poor practice and poor care (Scholes *et al.*, 2004).[1] However, Freshwater and Biley (2005: 15) caution that: 'caring is not necessarily the anti-thesis to modern nursing practice, but it is perhaps not so easily recognised or articulated in our rapidly changing health care environment'.

The Government's response to criticisms about standards of care has been a whole-hearted commitment to the modern matron role to raise standards of care (DH, 2002a); the Chief Nurse considered 'Essence of Care' a tool by which standards could be measured and practice development implemented to address the shortfalls identified (Mullally, 2001). In response to the criticisms, the RCN, the King's Fund, Unison and the Chief Nurse defended nursing, claiming that care is at the core of practice (Parish, 2003).

Analysis of the 'new' or 'partnership' pre-registration nursing curricula found that care was indeed espoused as the essence of nursing but students described how this had become something other when put into practice (Scholes *et al.*, 2004). The students (*N* = 232) interviewed for this study identified that their most powerful learning experiences originated in practice, and dis-missed teaching or demonstration of high standards of care within the college setting as part of the theory practice gap (ibid.). However, students did report that they had witnessed excellence in care, and these experiences tended to be in specialist areas where the ratio of staff to patients was greatly increased.

---

[1] The 'new' curriculum is known around the UK by three main names: *Making a Difference*, as it was in response to the Government's report on the contribution of nursing and midwifery (DH, 1999); competency-based curriculum in response to the Peach Report (UKCC, 1999), which identified that there was a need for the curriculum to be far more skills and competency based to enable newly qualified staff to be 'fit for purpose'; and finally by the Department of Health (DH) as the partnership curriculum as they saw that the key way forward to redress this apparent need was through closer partnership between HEIs and Trusts to create more effective learning environments in practice as well as in the academic setting. The DH commissioned a three-year evaluation undertaken by Scholes *et al.* (2004) that included all the 16 first-wave sites across the country. The data were derived from 71 hours' observation of practice and 177 hours shadowing students and their mentors, supplemented by a total of 848 interviews with clinicians, educationalists and education commissioners undertaken over a three-year period from December 2000 to July 2003.

Most, although not all, critical care settings were identified by the students as areas where they were *more likely* to be exposed to role models whose practice had care at the core (ibid.).

So what is meant by care? Why should this be presented as a picture of excellent practice? How has it become so elusive? To answer these questions we need first to map a model of what is meant by excellent care.

Roach (1987) has described five attributes of caring. They comprise conscience, commitment, competence, confidence and compassion. Comportment was subsequently added to describe the way nurses should behave. Paterson and Zderad (1988) state that this emerges from an intentional and authentic presence. Sadler (1997) moves this on to describe the nurse using presence to effect a transformational relationship. Nurses have in critical care been identified as using presence and proximity, stillness, total attention and engagement with the patient to alleviate distress and discomfort. In this way they are said to use themselves as therapeutic tools (Scholes, 1996). This has been linked to experience and expertise that can only be achieved when nurses have mastery over the environment and practice knowledge (Scholes and Moore, 1997). This is essential in order to free conscious attention to noticing, attending and presencing that might otherwise be taken up by the conscious assimilation, processing of information and formulation of those data into clinical judgements that occupy the conscious attention of less experienced nurses (Benner, 1984; Benner *et al.*, 1999). Thus expressions of caring can be made explicit within a technological environment; they are neither polarised nor paradoxical (Musk, 2004). Indeed, if this research were advanced and it could be demonstrated that the expert nurse's therapeutic presence could be used to substitute for sedation or analgesia, the argument for clinical nursing expertise at the bedside would be strengthened, especially in a highly technological environment. The notion that nurses might be substituted by technicians is completely contradicted because nursing expertise is crucial to differentiate when the use of self can be effective and where medication and other interventions are essential (Scholes, 1996).

Excellent care cannot be separated from competent care. In this instance, competence refers to the knowledge that underpins the professional interventions that have been deliberately selected and delivered thoughtfully and with compassion (Benner, 1984; Benner and Wrubel, 1989; Benner *et al.*, 1996, 1999). It is affective, cognitive and behavioural. It is highly skilled, and embedded in professional artistry and craft knowledge (Titchen and Higgs, 2001). It may seem obvious and simple. It may seem effortless. But sustaining that degree of attentiveness, will and intention to interact knowledgeably in such a way sets apart excellent care from lay care.

Sensitive and knowledgeable care is exemplified by the state of vigilance: the nurse being in a condition of readiness to respond to the needs of the patient. To do this the nurse needs to have a sound theoretical knowledge base which is readily applied, adapted and refined through experience, to the patient's situation. This requires thought beyond the moment, being alert to and recognising the patient's current and future needs and focusing on small things that make a considerable difference to them (McLeod, 1996). It is about fully engaging and thinking through, watching over and thinking for (when necessary) or with the patient (Benner *et al.*, 1999).

To help illustrate what I mean by excellent care I will provide a series of scenarios that compare and contrast examples of good with indifferent care. They have been provided to encourage the reader to critically reflect upon these situations and consider the situation from the patient's or relative's perspective.

Nurses, do not intentionally harm their patients, but they may do so in a cast-away gesture or word, a momentary lapse in concentration. In the first scenario, I reflect again on my experience as a trauma patient and on the impact of a staff nurse's initial contact with me.

Scenario 2.1:   Self before service

One night an agency nurse walked into my room, held his head to one side, lifted his hand and said: 'I know who you are and don't think I am either impressed or intimidated by that. You are one of 32 patients so don't expect any special favours.' I was scared. What if I needed his help that night? How could I possibly ask for his assistance? I could feel myself getting tearful and felt it important not to show my tears. There was no fear of that. He was closed off, shut down. I could feel myself tense, and with that the muscle spasm started, my fractures moved and the burning nerve pain began to build. This was going to be a long and painful night.

Maybe as nurses we can sympathise with a colleague setting out the ground rules and articulating their priorities. However, the manner in which this was done ultimately caused more work because I then needed additional analgesia. However, there are many practitioners who 'don't get nursing'. They seem to simulate caring, or go through the motions without truly engaging with the patient (Rubin, 1996). This can be read in an instant. It is something in their eyes (Watt, 1996; Wright and Sayre-Adams, 2005). Some completely avoid eye contact; others might superficially glance at you and then away. Some give the impression that you are viewed with suspicion, a burden that gets in the way of what they are doing. You lie there unnoticed outside their gaze, helpless and vulnerable. You feel too ill at ease to ask for anything for fear this will alienate or distance them further. You are set in a position of deference, feeling a nuisance, 'more work' rather than the very reason why they are there in the first place.

Scenario 2.2:   The impact of a cast-away comment

When the attending trauma doctor assessed me in casualty, he introduced himself but I could not catch his name. I was disorientated by the trauma and the vast amounts of analgesia used to ease my transfer from the ground on to a stretcher, into the helicopter, to the ambulance, on arrival in A&E, and for transfer from stretcher to trolley. One of my strongest memories of that day was how many times I was moved. Each movement was agony, creating a sensation that my pelvis was opening up like a chocolate orange, segmented, broken. I felt as though I had come undone. Turning set off a cycle of muscle spasm, bone movement and severe nerve pain. At this stage, I could not find the words to describe it. Instead the pain found expression through a low guttural moan that leaked from under my diaphragm and spilled out from my mouth. I would will myself to push that sound back, but it had started and could not be caught. This clearly irritated the doctor who said: 'Julie, be quiet. We are only trying to assess you. Where does it hurt? What is wrong?'

I was a member of staff. By dint of my background I was supposed to be informed and to provide detailed, sensible information. My brain could not compute or function. My tongue was tied, I could not find the words to describe that pain, locate it or control my response to it. It consumed me as it blurred my consciousness. I was held in contempt for having made the mistake of falling from a horse: injuring myself at leisure, consuming the staff's valuable time with my self-inflicted wounds. I felt a 'rubbish patient' (Jeffrey, 1979) and seriously doubted the legitimacy of my attendance in A&E. I wanted to be stoic, but stoicism escaped me. I was terrified.

Scenario 2.3:   Contrasting absence and presence

Throughout my time in A&E I had a profound sense that I was falling. I felt that I would drop from the trolley, and I wanted the cot side in place to stop me from falling. The sister was in the trauma room busying herself with my property. I lifted my hand towards her and this small pathetic voice (to my shock it was *my* voice) said, 'Please, sister, stop me from falling.' She put my hand back down to my side, pulled up the trolley side and returned to her task.

A staff nurse came into the trauma room. She took my hand. She locked into me – made me feel safe. She busied herself with the observations, but she kept me constantly in her gaze. She was concerned and took my distress seriously. She promised to fetch more analgesia. All too soon I lost my empathic carer. We were separated as I was sent round to X-ray.

For me that staff nurse demonstrated **care** of a trauma patient. She was sensitive and kind. She stopped for a moment to take my hand. She noticed and empathically considered the physical, psychological and social discomfort that this sudden transition had brought about. She watched over me, was there beside me, with me, concerned, attentive. She noticed my situation, responded to that, and generously gave something of herself. And however brief, in that moment I felt understood and well protected.

> **Scenario 2.4:   A model of excellence**
>
> Fourteen days later, I was visited by the pain team who were the most magnificent practitioners. Their opening remark as they took my hand was: 'I hear you have had the most dreadful time.'[2] They legitimised my situation and made me feel I was not unduly making a fuss. They were here to solve the problems. They could do something to help me heal. They gave me control through the patient-controlled analgesia (PCA). They listened. They were thoughtful. They were genuinely present. They had a wealth of knowledge and applied that to get on top of the pain and try out different medications to cap it. They talked through their decision making, involved me and shared their ideas. They gave me their time. They smiled. They were warm. I wasn't rubbish. They were pleased to help me and use their skilled professional artistry to confidently intervene. At last I felt someone had stopped me from falling.

When I reflect on why this was excellent practice, I conclude that it is because: (a) it was knowledgeable, informed and considered; (b) that was what I needed as a patient; and (c) it was so rare. These experiences are now compared with the findings in the literature to construct a model of caring excellence.

Self in therapeutic service

Presence or being attentive to the patient (Benner, 1984; Tanner *et al.*, 1993) is central to any construct of care. To do this, the nurse needs to set aside 'mental busy-ness' (Wright and Sayre-Adams, 2005: 14), and be beside someone as an 'uncluttered self' (ibid.: 15). Such presence creates a relaxation response in the patient. The converse is true in the absence of a present nurse as depicted in scenarios 2–3 above. However, to maintain this level of commitment and intentionality in the interaction requires the nurse to be self-aware, and to acknowledge when her inner resources are running out and find ways to restore them (Salvage, 2004).

Fundamentally, interactions of this kind require energy (Faugier, 2005), an investment of self to be other-serving (Gallagher, 2005). It is something linked to expert practice and experience, because it happens at a point where the professional and personal self fuse in a genuine expression of care. It is not a self-less act, but it is not selfish. Expert practitioners who interact in this way are rewarded by the fact that their interactions have a therapeutic outcome. The patient is put at ease and feels confident in the space of the interaction, the tension eases, and healing can take place. Healing in this instance refers to the release of intense emotions, physical tension or psychological turmoil which impede healing at a biological or cellular level (Wright and Sayre-Adams,

---

[2] I had been discharged home after 24 hours to 'self care' as the long-term treatment was bed rest. On orthopaedic review 10 days post injury, I was immediately admitted for pain management and full nursing care.

2005). It also opens the opportunity to fully engage with the patient, to actively listen and hear what is said (Butterworth, 2004). At this point deliberative interventions to continue to support that person can be initiated. The process of itself sustains further commitment to practise in this way.

The therapeutic milieu that is created and the dignity and respect of the interaction amount to far more than the sum of the parts. They can be created in an instant, the moment may be transitory, but the impact on the patient or their relative is powerful beyond measure. This does require the nurse to be motivated, intentional and willing to give in this way (Wright and Sayre-Adams, 2005). It situates the nurse in a position of providing a service which is patient centred, respectful and holistic (Kitson, 2004) and where the nurse uses self as the therapeutic tool (McMahon and Pearson, 1991).

Magnet (2003) concluded from her experience that the concept of nursing as doing service for others has been lost. The term 'service' conjures up images of self-sacrifice and submission which run counter to contemporary society and indeed the ethos of the profession today (Salvage, 2004). However, deliberative, thoughtful care based on the central premise of using self as a therapeutic tool fundamentally shifts the notion of doing a service for someone to being beside someone and working with them to achieve healing. This is further assisted by considering nursing to be about alleviating suffering (Eriksson, 1995), and to do this is the 'privileged place of nursing' (Benner and Wrubel, 1989: xi). To illustrate this privilege I have drawn upon a reflective account of recent experience whilst in clinical practice.

Scenario 2.5: Cure and care

On a recent return to clinical practice, I worked beside a highly intelligent, enthusiastic doctor undertaking the critical care rotation. He had been involved in the resuscitation of Arthur, an 86-year-old man who had very suddenly developed sepsis. The full sepsis protocol was implemented, including starting activated protein C, on the basis that he was fit and well prior to this sudden illness. A number of highly invasive interventions were made by Dr Smith under the supervision of the intensivist. Despite increasing the inotropes up to the maximum dose, this had little effect on Arthur's blood pressure. Likewise, the introduction of nitric oxide to the ventilatory circuit made little or no impact on his PO_2 levels. The relatives were consulted. They agreed that further efforts to prolong his life were futile, and the decision to withdraw was made. As if with a sigh of relief, Arthur died almost instantly. But a lasting memory was seeing Dr Smith slumped in front of the central computer screen, heavy head in hands staring at the monitor watching Arthur's physiological parameters fade away. He was clearly pained by this experience and when a supportive gesture and word were shared, he said: 'It's just so hard. We are not here to watch people die. I feel so hopeless.' I wanted to urge him not to watch the computer, but sit beside the patient and hold his hand and be beside him in his dying. Instead I found myself uttering the platitude: 'Sometimes it is kinder to let people go, especially when the outcome is so inevitable.'

This example serves as a potent reminder of how nurses work differently with the patient. It would be strange indeed to find a doctor sitting beside someone as they died, but not so a nurse. Therein lies the most privileged position of nursing: being beside people, alleviating suffering, making decisions about patients based upon objective scientific facts but tempered by the experience of providing intimate, purposeful care even if this is to ease them towards a dignified death (Henderson, 1960). The difference lies in the proximity to the patient, what we do, when we do it and over a period of time that allows us to build channels of communication even with deeply unconscious patients and their relatives (Williams, 2003). Such is the gift of nursing and how it enables us to define hopelessness in quite different terms from those that apply for the medical profession. When cure stops, care continues, and this left Dr Smith staring sadly at the screen watching his patient die. What strength and courage are needed to stand beside someone who dies! The emotional labour (Hochschilds, 1983; Smith, 1992) of one I suspect is no greater than the emotional labour of the other, but how much more can you do when you keep caring rather than position yourself behind a screen and stare on in hopelessness?

Seeing nursing as a privileged position fundamentally alters the way in which nurses interact with their patients and opens new possibilities for both. Disparaging views of nursing as low paid, stigmatic, routinised, unpleasant and temporary employment before gaining a satisfying job can only inhibit functioning in a therapeutic way (Wright and Sayre-Adams, 2005). However, within British nursing, there are a number of practising nurses who come to work each day with such resentment and baggage (Norris, 2000). Students who took part in the partnership evaluation identified not infrequent exposure to such ideas from their mentors (Scholes *et al.*, 2004). Although rejecting such messages, the students said that, when they encountered it, they could not help but pick up on the contagion of negativity (ibid.). I suspect the agency nurse described in the first scenario was one of them. Magnet (2003) certainly experienced their lack of care.

It is the little things that count (McLeod, 1994), but it is these little things that make a staggering difference to the patient's experience. The following example is one drawn from observation as a researcher. In this scenario, the nurse seems shut down to seeing the obvious. The discussion expands to consider the way in which technical, rational information and the softer aspects of nursing merge to demonstrate an alternative but high quality interaction with the patient.

Scenario 2.6:   Caring as common sense

A highly technically competent nurse was observed interacting with three high dependency unit (HDU) patients. One patient had an extremely high temperature and was florid, dry and clearly unwell. The nurse had recorded the temperature, rushed off and collected a fan, set this off at the fastest rate and moved on to the next patient. The nurse had failed to remove the blanket off the patient and replace this with a cool sheet. She had not considered offering a cool drink or ice to sip (even though the patient was not nil by mouth), nor a tepid sponge although clearly the patient could have benefited from any one if not all of these interventions. Shortly after this she contacted the doctor and reported the pyrexia and suggested blood cultures might be taken.

The most powerfully obvious, common sense solution to this situation would have been to remove the blanket, but the nurse had either simply not noticed this or was so intent on the equation: pyrexia > 40°C = fan + blood cultures that she was blinkered.

Has the quest for hard evidence diminished our capacity to attend to the softer aspects of nursing (Gallagher, 2005)? The stark reality is that the nurse did not offer the patient any intervention to make him feel comfortable. A fan blowing hard into the face is not comforting, nor is it as effective as tepid sponging (Nicol *et al.*, 2004) or ice cooling in hyper-pyrexia (Smith, 2005). Offering ice to suck or a cold drink, turning a pillow over to the cool side, or placing a cold flannel behind the neck, may do little to reduce the temperature, but would do a lot to make the patient more comfortable. It would create the opportunity for attentive presence, engagement and demonstration of genuine concern. Furthermore, this interaction would do much to relax the patient and help alleviate their distress.

If you had seen the nurse take all these actions, probably in an effortless, swift yet calm manner, you would draw the conclusion that she was an excellent and professionally mature nurse. You might also have noted that the excellent nurse would have delegated to the health care assistant (HCA) the task of bleeping the doctor and choose to make the nursing interventions herself so she might more thoroughly undertake a full physical assessment of the patient (especially as there was another registered nurse present on the HDU to monitor the other patients). Such priorities would be based on patient need, rather than on any sense of what might be considered bureaucratic, or hierarchical delegation. Thus the nurse would have demonstrated flexibility, situational discrimination and a deliberate choice to be at the bedside, because she recognised and could justify this as the greater need for the patient at the time: all markers of expertise (Benner *et al.*, 1996). She would remain alert and watchful, responsive to need, delivering care which would reward her with more knowledge against which she could inform her interactions (Benner *et al.*, 1999). There is a positive feedback loop that would sustain her attentiveness and will to deliver care of the highest standard, and she would be rewarded by the fact that she had delivered care well (Scholes and Moore, 1997).

To do this requires there to be skills, dexterity and mastery of practice knowledge and the therapeutic environment, combined with a healthy dose of common sense (Scholes, 1996). Or, perhaps as McLeod (1994) pointed out, 'uncommonly common sense'. To be safe, the practitioner has to know:

when to interact and when to watchfully wait; and what to delegate and when, without prejudicing the safety of that patient or any others. Even in this simple scenario, with apparently simple solutions, the wealth of practice knowledge and experiential wisdom that differentiates good practice from bad, excellent from good is remarkable. What is perhaps more remarkable is that it often goes unstated and sadly unwitnessed by students. Thus the invaluable impact of role modelling these behaviours is lost to successive generations of nurses.

Maybe the nurse in the scenario felt too hard pressed for time to invest in such acts of caring but, if hard pressed, why didn't the nurse feel able to delegate the tepid sponge to the HCA or ask her to offer a cool drink or ice to the patient? Even if we shift to analyse the technical rationale of actions taken, they fail to meet the fundamental need of comfort. Why did she not check the drug chart for antipyretics and time of administration? If not charted, why did she not request this from the doctor at the same time as the request for blood cultures? In this context, the pyrexia might be addressed alongside making the patient feel more comfortable.

All of us have had a pyrexia at some point in our lives, and have experience of what we did to make ourselves comfortable. What then has obstructed the experiential from impacting upon the act of caring in this scenario? Is it deference to hard science in a dominant culture that requires all interventions to be evidence based (Freshwater and Biley, 2005)? Has this happened as we struggle to shake off images of subservience or even 'dirty work' (Salvage, 2004), or simply through a desire to pursue the technical to evidence our knowledge and skill (Gallagher, 2005)? Is this an example of being 'too posh to wash' (BBC, 2005) or too clever to care (Gallagher, 2005)? Or have we become so engrossed in the mantra of being busy that we busily engage in time-consuming actions that have nothing to do with immediate care delivery (Melia, 1981)?

Factors that impede caring excellence

What factors have subjugated the core values of nursing and made them seem so special when they are in evidence? How has nursing become infiltrated by people with low morale and without a commitment to the enterprise of caring, and who undervalue the profession? Of course this is multifactorial (Williams *et al.*, 2003). Some of the factors will be examined to consider how these potential barriers might be overcome to achieve excellence in caring by the majority, not, sadly as seems to be the current case, the minority.

Context

The volume of patients and clients the modern health service has to manage continues to grow. At the same time, rapid advances in health care technologies and an ageing population have contributed to higher patient dependency. All this has taken place in the context of shifting social, political and economic patterns. The public is better informed and has higher expectations of the health care service (Weinstein, 1996). In response to this, workforce reconfigurations have placed new demands upon practitioners and have changed the way we work with patients and clients (Parkin, 1995). A decade ago, Richardson and Maynard (1995) estimated that 30% of doctors could be replaced by nurses. Following a literature review they found that authors estimated between 30 and 70% of the tasks performed by doctors could be carried out by nurses, representing a considerable cost saving to the NHS (ibid.).

The need for the reconfiguration of services and changing workforce pattern (DH 2002b) has been heralded by a number of changes. The reduction in junior doctors' hours (DH, 1991) and more recently the European Working Time Directive (The Working Time (Amendment) Regulations 2003) have required a significant review of how competencies and skills can be shared or blended across the multidisciplinary team to accommodate the changes in doctors' working hours (Albarran and Scholes, 2005). Fundamentally, nursing has absorbed many of the new models of working, through the inception of 'blended' roles whereby aspects of practice traditionally delivered by different disciplines (mainly doctors) have been amalgamated to provide a service based on patient need and timely provision (Adam, 2004). However, all this is set in the context of a major shortfall in NHS personnel to meet health care demand, hence the need to consider alternative approaches to provision and increase flexibility in deploying the workforce (NHS Modernisation Agency, 2003). The net result has been major reconsideration of who does what, when and how. As nurses undertake more advanced, expanded or blended roles, they in turn need to delegate aspects of care (Albarran and Scholes, 2005). The technicians or health care assistants who carry out delegated nursing tasks may neither have worked closely with nor have been supervised directly by practitioners of caring excellence. This has contributed to the reduced likelihood of core values being realised in everyday practice.

Factors that impede the transmission of expertise

Two recent studies have found that students identified that they spent little time working directly with qualified staff on the ward (Duffy, 2003; Scholes *et al.*, 2004). Even when they did, they had to compete with a variety of other students each vying for the attention of the mentor. Many described working alongside agency staff, and newly registered students from adaptation courses, who might know little about the course and priorities for clinical learning for the student on that placement. In this situation, the student might find themselves guiding the mentor (Duffy, 2003; Scholes *et al.*, 2004).

The pre-registration students saw the role of the permanent staff nurse to be about managing the ward, liaising with other agencies and health care professionals, drug administration, setting up IVs and the like. Rarely did they see staff nurses providing fundamental care; they perceived this to be the domain of the HCAs. Many had undertaken this role to gain health care experience prior to being accepted on the programme, and were keen to distance themselves from that and concentrate on acquiring the skills to fit them for what they considered the qualified role to be about. Thus they placed little value on seeking out fundamental care experiences as important learning opportunities (Scholes *et al.*, 2004). In such circumstances the net result has been the degradation in value of fundamental caring skills and a reluctance to emphasise their importance to the students they subsequently supervise once they are qualified.

The updraft of excellent practitioners into specialist roles (minimum requirement 5 years' post-registration experience and 2 years in the speciality before being awarded the post (Trent Cancer Nurses Allied Health Professions Advisory Group, 2001)) means that patients are not exposed to, and students do not necessarily witness, high quality fundamental care provision and expert practice round the clock. If they do observe the care of a specialist, this is viewed as episodic and different. Ultimately this leads to the continuous dilution of high quality provision as more experienced and excellent carers take up specialist roles that befit their talent. But their upward mobility creates a vacuum in experience and excellence which cannot easily be filled, especially in a recruitment crisis. Further, the retention crisis and high vacancy factor have done much to damage morale (Williams *et al.*, 2003) and this inevitably impacts upon the quality of the therapeutic provision.

This is a critical factor that mentors in critical care environments need to consider: first to demonstrate and make these skills absolutely explicit when they work with pre-registration students on their unit. Secondly, when newly qualified staff come to critical care environments, preceptors may find they need to assess each novice's fundamental care skills and stress their importance, especially as the novice may feel the need to focus solely on the new technology in the environment (Scholes and Smith, 1997).

The building profile of factors that impede caring excellence cannot omit a painful truth: that nursing is populated by some practitioners who are not interested in being nurses. The issues identified above have explored how the interest might have been extinguished through socialisation or lack of a positive role model. However, there is a growing concern that recruits now enter nursing with an entirely different set of expectations and with a non-vocational purpose (Salvage, 2004).

Nurses who are uninterested in nursing

The changing demographic, social and economic climate has resulted in the NHS having to compete directly for potential recruits with other public sector and associated employers (HM Treasury, 2002). The target set by the Government[3] to recruit more nurses to meet the demands of the NHS has left some with a concern that nursing is becoming populated by people who are uninterested in nursing.

The most significant route to expansion has been planned through increasing pre-registration commissions. A number of initiatives have been set in place to increase the numbers of students including: attracting mature entrants,[4] widening the entry gate, offering as much flexibility as possible through stepping on and off the programme, HCA sponsorship and offering accelerated pathways towards registration (DH, 1999). All these strategies were intent on attracting suitable people to nursing, especially those with life experiences that could enhance their potential as carers. However, selecting suitable candidates while meeting recruitment targets remains a tension (Scholes *et al.*, 2004). Clinicians and academics were concerned that candidates who might previously have been rejected were given the benefit of the doubt and offered a place on the programme because of the increased commissioning for students. Trusts and higher education institutions (HEIs) are increasingly concerned to ensure that poor quality practitioners are selected out of the programme before registration and employment. They felt a certain level of attrition should be considered healthy as it demonstrates rigour in the professional quality assurance procedures within the HEI (ibid.). However, clinical and academic participants expressed concern that, as long as HEIs are faced with financial penalties for attrition rates over 13% (DH, 2002c), some unsuitable nurses would continue to end up in practice (Scholes *et al.*, 2004). Unsuitability was described as 'inappropriate attitude', 'uncaring', 'closed off', 'lacking commitment' and 'disinterested': the antithesis of therapeutic presence. What impact does this have on students when their mentors perceive current practice to be a 'battle zone' (Norris, 2000: 133)?

Qualified staff described how they had become this way as a result of their fatigue from struggling to resolve organisational issues in general wards related to staffing levels and skill mix, or from managing conflict that can arise between different staff groups and sometimes patients and their relatives. This evoked feelings of being scared, stressed and unsupported, highly exposed to criticism and in the 'line of fire', and resulted in low morale and chronic fatigue. Three categories of nurses emerged: the 'battle weary', the 'battle hardened'

---

[3] The Government target to increase the number of qualified nurses by 20 000 by 2004 (DH, 1999) was achieved one year ahead of schedule. Work has been undertaken to attract more nurses back to the NHS following a career break and by recruiting significant numbers of overseas staff (16 155 overseas nurses joined the register in 2002: NMC, 2002) to address the vacancy factor, with the Prime Minister announcing that 50 000 new nurses had been recruited since 1997 (DH, 2003). However, the estimated number of nurses, midwives and HVs that will be needed by 2008 has increased to 35 000 (HM Treasury, 2002). These data pre-date the latest financial crisis whereby nursing staff are being made redundant or newly qualified nurses do not get jobs (Hansard, 24/5/2006).

[4] The mean age of adult student respondents was 31.16; and for mental health (MH) the mean age of students was 33.45 (Third Students Survey, Robinson and Hill, 2003), with 41% stating they had caring responsibilities outside the course (38% adult and 49% MH respondents: IES Third Student Survey: ibid.).

and the 'survivors'.[5] Nurses seemed to vacillate between these categories depending on the experiences of the day. Importantly, one coping strategy was by 'switching off' and 'getting through the shift' (Norris, 2000). This level of disengagement and the impact of such role models on the student population becomes a self-replicating cycle of spiralling negativity: one which stands little chance, if it goes unchecked, of enabling them to realise their potential as excellent carers.

The challenge for preceptors and managers is to see if these practitioners can be facilitated to make a transition which effects a more positive outlook and opens the potential for them to practise in a therapeutic way and cope more effectively within existing organisational constraints. Such an approach would require a considerable investment, but might ultimately have a positive impact on retention (see Chapters 6 and 7 for strategies to deal with these situations). However, some practitioners may be so uninterested in nursing that no investment can enable them to change their attitude. In these instances, their departure from the profession can only be encouraged to minimise 'negativity contamination' and, of paramount importance, to limit the potential damage they cause the patient.

Finally, core values cannot exist in a vacuum, and although the wider societal and cultural expectations are changing, practitioners are also exposed to significant cultural dynamics within the NHS. Although not essentially paradoxical, there can be a tension between the realisation of core nursing values when set in the context of a culture that values efficiency and effectiveness. So the final discussion, which focuses on the barriers to realise excellence in care, has to address the impact of managerialism and marketisation.

Managerialism and marketisation

The dominance of managerialism in the NHS gained hold in the 1980s following Griffiths' inquiry on management of the NHS (Griffiths, 1983). This heralded the introduction of business principles to influence the way in which health care was delivered. Within this technical rational model the primary motivation shifted to one of managed systems to enhance efficiency and effectiveness (Smart, 1999). Thus the philanthropic ideals of the NHS have shifted to values that venerate productivity, standardisation, predictability and control (Smart, 1999). This has been termed the McDonaldization of health care and education (Ritzer, 1996) (see Chapter 5). However, it is mentioned here because many of the systems set in place to quality-assure, risk-manage,

---

[5] Norris (2000) found more survivors amongst the participants who worked in critical care environments. She concluded this was the case because they had greater control and autonomy in the care of their patients than staff on acute care wards, where the nurses perpetually struggled to provide care in a constantly changing environment of multiple and competing demands.

standardise, enhance predictability and so forth demand extensive documentation. Thus systems set in place to enhance efficiency and effectiveness do much to distance practitioners from the patient and occupy their time with paperwork or computer returns. Although there is great political will to reduce the paperwork in the NHS and replace this with efficient computer systems, a number of large-scale IT initiatives have failed, exacerbating administrative delays (NHS Executive, 1998). Furthermore, targets for surgical admissions, length of stay, time lapse from referral to treatments, etc. have shifted the emphasis and altered the mind set of practitioners. In addition, the drive for evidence to inform health care delivery has the potential to overwhelm individual expression of caring (Freshwater and Biley, 2005). Thus the art of nursing and medicine (time consuming, unpredictable and non-standardised) falls victim to the more pressing agenda of efficiency and effectiveness.

As generations of practitioners foster the business attitude, core values seem a whimsical fancy, a brush with the past out of step with today's modern NHS. However, there does seem to be a genuine renaissance in caring values (for example, the Nursing Standards Core Values Series, 2004–5), resulting, not least, from the consumer voice and public outcry about declining standards of care in the NHS (e.g. Magnet, 2003; Sergent, 2003; Dispatches, Channel 4: 31 January 2005). The next great challenge is to deliver efficiency and effectiveness with excellence in care at the core.

In the next chapter Caroline Williams reviews the policies and political will that drive the modernisation agenda, and the impact this has had on critical care provision.

References

Adam S (2004) Plugging the gap – critical care skills are the current universal commodity. *Nursing in Critical Care* **9**(5): 195–198.

Albarran J and Scholes J (2005) Blurred, blended or disappearing – the image of critical care nursing. Editorial, *Nursing in Critical Care* **10**(1): 1–3.

BBC (2005) News UK Edition Nurses cannot be too posh to wash. http//news.bbc.co.uk/1/hi/health/3701855.stm (accessed 5 January 2005).

Benner P (1984) *From Novice to Expert: Excellence and Power in Clinical Nursing*. Menlo Park, CA: Addison-Wesley.

Benner P and Wrubel J (1989) *The Primacy of Caring. Stress and Coping in Health and Illness*. Menlo Park, CA: Addison-Wesley.

Benner P, Tanner C and Chesla C (1996) *Expertise in Nursing Practice: Caring, Clinical Judgement and Ethics*. New York: Springer.

Benner P, Hooper-Kyriakidis P and Stannard D (1999) *Clinical Wisdom and Interventions in Critical Care: A Thinking-in-action Approach*. Philadelphia, WB Saunders.

Butterworth T (2004) Lend me your ears. *Nursing Standard* **19**(13): 16–17.

Department of Health (1991) Hours of work of doctors in training the New Deal. London, DH (executive letter: EL(91) 82).

Department of Health (1999) *Making a Difference, Strengthening the Nursing, Midwifery and Health Visiting Contribution to Health and Healthcare*. London: DH.

Department of Health (2002a) *Modern Matrons in the NHS: a Progress Report*. London: DH.

Department of Health (2002b) *Changing Workforce Programme. New Ways of Working in Health Care*. London: DH.

Department of Health (2002c) *Recruitment and Progression – Minimising Attrition from NHS-funded Pre-registration Healthcare Courses* www.dh.gov.uk/assetRoot/04/07/16/31/04071631.pdf (accessed 18 January 2005).

Department of Health (2002d) *Liberating the Talents: Helping Primary Care Trusts to Deliver the NHS Plan*. London: The Stationery Office.

Department of Health (2003) *Further Increases in Numbers of Nurses and Doctors Working in the NHS*. http://www.dh.gov.uk/PublicationsAndStatistics/PressReleases/PressReleasesNotices/fs/en?CONTENT_ID=4047268&chk=bZbHnn. Accessed 19 April 2006.

Department of Health (2004) *The NHS Knowledge and Skills Framework (NHS KSF) and the Development Review Process*. London: DH.

Duffy K (2003) *Failing Students: A Qualitative Study of Factors that Influence the Decisions Regarding the Assessment of Students' Competence to Practise*. Glasgow: Caledonian Nursing and Midwifery Research Centre, Glasgow Caledonian University.

Eriksson K (1995) *Det Lidende Menneske* [The suffering human being] Copenhagen: Munsgaard.

Faugier J (2005) Reality check. *Nursing Standard* **19**(19): 14–15.

Freshwater D and Biley F (2005) Heart of the matter. *Nursing Standard* **19**(20): 14–15.

Gallagher A (2005) Too clever to care? *Nursing Standard* **19**(18): 14–15.

Griffiths R (1983) *Report of the NHS Management Inquiry*. London: Department of Health and Social Security.

Hansard (24/5/2006) *Nuring*. www.publications.parliament.uk/pa/cm200506/cmhansrd/cm060524/halltext/60524h0105.htm.

Henderson V (1960) *Basic Principles of Nursing*. Geneva: International Council of Nurses.

HM Treasury (2002) *Cost Cutting Review of the Labour Market*. London: HM Treasury.

Hochschilds A (1983) *The Managed Heart: Commercialisation of Human Feeling*. Berkeley, CA: University of California Press.

Jeffrey R (1979) Normal rubbish: deviant patients in casualty departments. *Sociology of Health and Illness* **1**(1): 90–107.

Kitson A (2004) The whole person. *Nursing Standard* **19**(12): 14–15.

McLeod M (1994) It's the little things that count: the hidden complexity of everyday clinical nursing practice. *Journal of Clinical Nursing* **3**: 361–368.

McLeod M (1996) *Practising Nursing – Becoming Experienced*. New York: Churchill Livingstone.

Magnet J (2003) Witness: What's wrong with nursing? *Prospect* December 2003.

McMahon R and Pearson A (1991) *Nursing as Therapy*. London: Chapman & Hall.

Melia K (1981) Student nurses' accounts of their work and training: a qualitative analysis. Unpublished PhD Thesis, Edinburgh.

Mullally S (2001) *The Essence of Care, Patient-focused Benchmarking for Health Care Practitioners*. London: DH, Office of the Chief Nurse.

Musk A (2004) Proficiency with technology and the expression of caring: can we reconcile these polarised views? *International Journal of Human Caring* **8**(2): 13–19.

NHS Executive (1998) *Information for Health: an Information Strategy for the Modern NHS*. London: DH.

NHS Modernisation Agency (2003) *New Ways of Working*. http://www.modern.nhs.uk/scripts/default.asp?siet_id=47 (accessed 15 August 2004).

Nicol M, Bavin C, Bedford Turner S, Cronin P and Rawlings-Anderson K (2004) *Essential Nursing Skills*, 2nd Edition. Edinburgh: Mosby.

Norris M (2000) Contextual factors that enable or disable nurses' professional practice. Unpublished DPhil Thesis, University of Sussex.

Nursing and Midwifery Council (NMC) (2002) *NMC Register Statistics*. NMC press release, May.

Parish C (2003) Nurses defend care after professionalism is attacked. *Nursing Standard* **8**(12).

Parkin P (1995) Nursing the future: a re-examination of the professionalisation thesis in the light of some recent developments. *Journal of Advanced Nursing* **21**: 561–567.

Paterson L and Zderad P (1988) *Humanistic Nursing*. New York: League for Nursing Press.

Richardson G and Maynard A (1995) *Fewer Doctors? More Nurses? A Review of the Knowledge Base of Doctor–Nurse Substitution*. Discussion Paper 135. York: The University of York Centre for Health Economics, York Health Economics Consortium, NHS Centre for Reviews and Dissemination.

Ritzer G (1996) *The McDonaldization of Society: An Investigation into the Changing Character of Contemporary Life*. Thousand Oaks, CA: Pine Forge.

Roach S (1987) *The Human Act of Caring*. Ottawa, Canadian Hospital Association.

Robinson D and Hill D (2003) *Evaluation of Nursing Education Partnership. Third Year Student Survey Final Report*. Brighton: Institute for Employment Studies.

Rubin J (1996) Impediments to the development of clinical knowledge and ethical judgement in critical care nursing. In Benner P, Tanner C and Chesla C (eds). *Expertise in Nursing Practice: Caring, Clinical Judgement and Ethics*. New York: Springer.

Sadler J (1997) Defining professional nurse caring: a triangulated study. *International Journal of Human Caring* **1**(3): 12–21.

Salvage J (2004) The call to nurture. *Nursing Standard* **19**(10): 16–17.

Scholes J (1996) How the critical care nurse uses self to the patient's therapeutic benefit. *Nursing in Critical Care* **1**(2): 60–66.

Scholes J and Moore M (1997) *Making a Difference: the Way in Which the Nurse Interacts with the Critical Care Environment and Uses Herself as a Therapeutic Tool*. ITU NDU Occasional Paper Series Number 2, University of Brighton [ISBN 1 87196679 5].

Scholes J and Smith M (1997) *Starting Afresh: the Impact of the Critical Care Milieu on Newcomers and Novices*. ITU NDU Occasional Paper Series Number 1, University of Brighton [ISBN 1 87 196692 2].

Scholes J, Freeman F, Gray M, Wallis B, Robinson D, Matthews-Smith G and Miller C (2004) *Evaluation of Nurse Education Partnerships*. www.brighton.ac.uk/inam/research/projects/partnerships_report.pdf.

Sergent H (2003) *Managing Not to Manage – Management in the NHS. The Story of Failure at the Heart of British Hospitals*. London: Centre for Policy Studies.

Smart B (1999) *Resisting McDonaldization*. London: Sage.

Smith J (2005) *Cooling Treatments*. www.chclibrary.org/micormed/0043820.html (accessed 18 January 2005).

Smith P (1992) *The Emotional Labour of Nursing. How Nurses Care*. London: Macmillan.

Tanner C, Benner P, Chesla C and Gordon D (1993) The phenomenology of knowing a patient. *Image* **25**(4): 273–280.

Titchen A and Higgs J (2001) A dynamic framework for the enhancement of health professional practice in an uncertain world: the practice–knowledge interface. In

Higgs J and Titchen A (eds). *Practice Knowledge and Expertise in the Health Professions.* Oxford: Butterworth Heinemann.

Trent Cancer Nurses Allied Health Professions Advisory Group (2001) *Nurse Specialists, Nurse Consultants, Nurse Leads: the Development and Implementation of New Roles to Improve Cancer and Palliative Care. An Advisory Report.* Trent Nurse Executive.

UKCC (1999) *Fitness for Practice.* London: United Kingdom Central Council for Nursing, Midwifery and Health Visiting.

Watt B (1996) *Patient: the True Story of a Rare Illness.* Harmondsworth: Penguin Books.

Weinstein J (1996) Sharing common professional problems – report from the UCET Autumn 1995 conference. *Journal of Professional Care* **10**(2): 195–197.

Working Time (Amendment) Regulations 2003. London: HMSO [ISBN 0110467523].

Williams C (2003) Nurse patient interaction in an intensive care setting. Unpublished PhD Thesis, University of Brighton.

Williams S, Coombs M and Lattimer V (2003) *Workforce Planning for Critical Care: a Rapid Review of the Literature (1990–2003)* www.modern.nhs.uk/criticalcare/5021/7117/Critical%20Care%20290503.pdf (accessed on 14 November 2004).

Wright S and Sayre-Adams J (2005) Encouraging nature to act. *Nursing Standard* **19**(1): 14–15.

Chapter 3

The dynamic context of critical care provision

Caroline Williams

Introduction

This chapter aims to highlight the key challenges and contextual dynamics that nurses face as they develop expertise within the field of critical care nursing. To do this it is important to consider briefly the influences that are driving change and modernisation currently within the National Health Service (NHS). The effects of this modernisation on critical care service provision will then be explored in relation to different areas of critical care practice, giving a brief glimpse of the diverse and numerous transitions which may impact on staff and patients alike. The final section explores workforce and education issues, both of which are central to improving staff satisfaction, retention and, ultimately, service delivery and patient care.

The NHS and the modernisation agenda

For over a decade, the NHS has been in the throes of rapid and constant change, perhaps even chaos (Ashworth, 2000). During these years, the NHS has been bombarded with demands for efficiency, cost cutting and a value-for-money service, a culture never before experienced by this public service provider (Coombs, 1999). With customer expectations and knowledge levels ever-rising, the health care team are required to provide a sound rationale for the care and treatment they provide (McSherry and Haddock, 1999), and to increase patient participation in both the planning and evaluation of health care provision (Department of Health (DH), 1992).

These initiatives were articulated clearly in the publication, *The NHS Plan*, published in July 2000. This was a radical, far-reaching plan of reform and investment to modernise the NHS over the subsequent 10 years. At the heart of the plan was a commitment to the needs of patients and clients in England, underpinned by the original principles of the NHS: '. . . the provision of quality care based on clinical need, irrespective of the patient's ability to pay, meeting the needs of people from all walks of life' (DH, 2000a). In 2004, the Government reported that investment in the NHS had grown from a budget of £33 billion to £67.4 billion, equating to a rise of over 50% per head of population (DH, 2004a).

The key challenges facing the NHS in 2000 were reported as a shortage of beds, across both acute and continuing care; significant shortfalls in appropriately qualified and experienced doctors and nurses; lengthy waiting times for both unscheduled and planned care; inadequate care for older people; and poor standards across hospital settings, particularly in relation to the cleanliness of wards and the facilities provided for patients and visitors within hospitals (DH, 2000a).

Over the past decade, the model of patient treatment and care has changed dramatically, with acute care in the community seeing rapid growth as day surgery and short-stay hospital admissions increase the workload for the community health care team (DH, 1999b). In-patient care has seen a comparable growth in the demand for more complex and technological care (Wigens and Westwood, 2000), with patients now cared for in hospital wards where they might once have required admission to high dependency or intensive care units (DH, 2000b). This pattern, commonly attributed to the United Kingdom's (UK) ageing population (DH, 1997c) and to technological advances (Atkinson, 1994), is reflected in community settings, where an increasing number of patients receive home-based treatment that 10–15 years ago would have been restricted to acute wards or high dependency units (HDUs), such as peritoneal dialysis or long-term parenteral and enteral nutrition.

Following the NHS Plan, the NHS Modernisation Agency was formed as the catalyst to bring this plan of change to reality, with the focus on improving patient care and patient services. To achieve this, the Modernisation Agency has formed partnerships with local and national private and public organisations within health and social care, with patients and carers, and with local NHS staff. The ethos that underpinned the Modernisation Agency's work was one through which change was facilitated rather than imposed, giving their partners the tools and confidence to engage in a process of ongoing improvement and evaluation. This programme of change did, however, have to ascribe to the key Principles of Modernisation, set out in somewhat overlapping guidelines, but which have become known as the Three Rs and the Five Simple Rules (see Table 3.1).

In critical care at this time, the demand for dedicated critical care services was growing steadily alongside the increasing acuity of patients admitted to hospital (Audit Commission, 1999; DH, 2000b). This was evidenced by a rise in the median number of beds within acute trusts' general intensive care units (ICUs) rising from four to six beds during 1993 to 1998 despite an overall drop in hospital beds over the same period (Audit Commission, 1999). This was followed by a 13% increase in the overall number of ICU beds in England and Wales between 1999 and 2002 (DH, 2002a).

Table 3.1 Principles of modernisation (from NHS Modernisation Agency, 2003a with permission of the Controller of HMSO. Crown copyright).

The Three Rs

- **Renewal:** More modern buildings and facilities, new equipment and information technology, more and better trained staff.
- **Redesign:** Services delivered in radically different ways with a much greater use of clinical networks to better co-ordinate services around the patient.
- **Respect:** A culture of mutual respect between politicians and the NHS, between different groups of staff and, crucially, between the NHS and those we serve.

The Five Simple Rules

(1) See things through the patient's eyes.
(2) Find a better way of doing things.
(3) Look at the whole picture.
(4) Give frontline staff the time and the tools to tackle the problems.
(5) Take small steps as well as big ones.

Defining critical care

Until the late 1990s, critical care was a term most often associated with discrete units, particularly ICUs, which were characterised by specially trained staff, higher staff–patient ratios, close observation and extensive technological monitoring (King's Fund, 1989). However, the changing nature and needs of patients being admitted to hospital indicated the need for a re-think. In 1999, following an extensive review of critical care services across the UK reported in *Critical to Success: The Place of Efficient and Effective Critical Care Services within the Acute Hospital* (Audit Commission, 1999), a perceptible change in focus was advocated, one in which critical care provision was driven by patient need and based on the *level* of care required by patients, and not on their location.

Critical care is care intended for patients who have the potential to recover, but for whom support and timely treatment are required if recovery has the chance to occur (Jennett, 1990). Critical care should therefore be regarded as a hospital-wide approach in which each patient has access to critical care, wherever they might be located. It should be seen as care that impacts on the patient's whole hospital experience, which may include care in some of the more discrete specialist units, such as the Accident and Emergency (A&E) department, the operating theatre, the ICU, or the coronary care unit (CCU), in addition to the care they receive within an acute ward. Thus the vision being advocated is one of 'critical care without walls' in which critical care is a *'comprehensive'* service driven by patient need (DH, 2000b).

Table 3.2 Classification of critical care patients based on patient need (from DH, 2000b with permission of the Controller of HMSO. Crown copyright).

Level 0:	Patients whose needs can be met through normal ward care in an acute hospital.
Level 1:	Patients at risk of deterioration, or those recently allocated from higher levels of care, whose needs can be met on an acute ward with additional advice and support from the critical care team.
Level 2:	Patients requiring more detailed observation or intervention including support for a single failing organ system or post-operative care, and those 'stepping down' from higher levels of care.
Level 3:	Patients requiring advanced respiratory support alone or basic respiratory support together with support for at least two organ systems. This level includes all complex patients requiring support for multi-organ failure.

Following this review of adult critical care services in the UK in 1999, the Audit Commission concluded that '*supply-side solutions*' where more critical care beds, and thus specialist nurses, were provided was not the sole answer (Audit Commission, 1999: 7). The report made a number of recommendations for increasing the effectiveness, and containing the spiralling cost, of intensive care services, and led to a further report from an expert group who were appointed by the Department of Health to develop a model for improving the delivery and organisation of critical services throughout the NHS in England (DH, 2000b).

Comprehensive Critical Care recommended that the existing categories used generally at that time to classify the severity of patients (i.e. 'ICU patient[1]' or 'HDU patient') be redefined into four levels of care (Table 3.2) based on the level of care patients needed (DH, 2000b).

By using this new system of classification, it was envisaged that the planning and provision of critical care services within trusts and across geographically located trusts would be more effective (DH, 2000b), enabling patients to be cared for in the most appropriate place, in a timely, effective manner which need not necessarily be in the most expensive or the most intensive location (Jennett, 1990), thus creating a picture of '*critical care without walls*' (DH, 2000b).

Modernising critical care services

In order to enact the programme of modernisation amongst critical care as outlined in *Comprehensive Critical Care* (DH, 2000b) and a subsequent strategy

---

[1] An 'ICU patient' would have been classified as such if admitted to the ICU (i.e. to a place), but may only have been admitted there if satisfactory or effective care was not available in an HDU or on a ward (Audit Commission, 1999).

for action document, *The Nursing Contribution to the Provision of Comprehensive Critical Care for Adults* (DH, 2001a), the NHS Modernisation Agency launched the Critical Care Programme in 2000, initially for 2 years but later extended until 2004.

Critical care networks

Central to this programme were the critical care networks. These networks, 29 in total, were established throughout England encompassing all trusts that provided critical care services (NHS Modernisation Agency, 2003b). Each network appointed a modernisation agency programme team to co-ordinate development activity. The aim was to promote improvements in the delivery, modernisation and management of services at local level whilst working collaboratively across networks to develop and share best practice in order to improve patient outcome and the patient's experience of critical care (DH, 2001a).

Change relating to service delivery and organisation of care was underpinned by the need to broaden the vision of critical care to encompass the needs of patients at risk of becoming critically ill, those who are critically ill and receiving critical care, and those who are recovering from critical illness (DH, 2001a). Through these collaborative networks, shared understanding of service requirements has led to marked improvements in analysing and reconfiguring patient pathways, with better access to services provided within this and across to other clinical networks such as coronary heart disease and cancer (NHS Modernisation Agency, 2003b). These networks have also played a significant part in the commissioning of critical care services, acting as a source of expert advice to commissioning teams. With advice available from across the networks as well as locally, commissioners of care can be better informed as to the appropriateness of their services to meet local need, whilst ensuring equity of provision in comparison with other regions (ibid.).

The chapter now turns to examine some of the practice developments in critical care that have emerged in response to the modernisation agenda.

Developments in critical care outreach

A central feature of modernisation in critical care that has been common to most networks is the development of critical care outreach services. Both the Audit Commission's review (1999) and the Department of Health's responses (DH, 2000b, 2001a) stated that outreach teams should have three aims:

- to enhance the early identification of patients whose condition is deteriorating in order to facilitate timely admission or avert the admission (or readmission) of patients to ICU;
- to facilitate discharge from ICU;
- to share critical care skills and knowledge with practitioners at ward level.

'Outreach' supports the philosophy of *critical care without walls* (DH, 2000b), and has been hailed as the new model of management for all patients with a need for critical care, no matter what their location. In the development of these teams, it has been acknowledged that the need for such a service was symptomatic of the increasing acuity of patients within acute hospital trusts, and the lack of an appropriately skilled workforce to meet such a demand (DH and NHS Modernisation Agency, 2003).

Some of the key service improvements reported since the introduction of outreach include:

- decrease in length of stay;
- reductions in the number of admissions and readmissions to critical care;
- reduced mortality rates;
- improvements in patient outcomes.

These reported outcomes (Coombs and Dillon, 2002; Ball *et al.*, 2003; Leary and Ridley, 2003; Pittard, 2003), whilst illustrating the potential benefits of this service, should be treated with some caution. Sound evidence to link the activities of outreach services to these improvements is still in its infancy, and further research[2] is needed to evaluate the implications of outreach not just from a critical perspective but also in relation to patient outcome and experience as a whole (DH and NHS Modernisation Agency, 2003).

That said, it could be argued that outreach has increased interaction between nurses, doctors and other allied health professionals (AHPs), such as physiotherapists, in critical care areas and those in acute wards, serving to break down some of the hidden barriers that may have hindered such valuable co-operation in the past. This outcome alone has the potential to impact positively on patient care. Furthermore, the inception of outreach teams has gone a considerable way towards facilitating another key target identified within the modernisation plan, namely the provision of competence-based high dependency training for all ward staff in acute hospitals by 2004 (DH, 2000b: 20). Whilst there is no single national model for the provision of outreach,[3] most teams offer education and training to staff in general wards and provide direct support at the bedside for varying periods. A concern voiced by some (Gibson, 1997; Smith, 2000) was that outreach would de-skill ward staff and introduce a further delay in patient management. Instead, outreach, in conjunction with training such as the ALERT (Acute Life-threatening Events: Recognition and Treatment) course (Smith *et al.*, 2002), has provided

---

[2] The Intensive Care National Audit & Research Centre commenced a study of outreach services in July 2004. This study, 'Evaluation of outreach services in critical care', aims to undertake a rigorous, scientific evaluation of outreach services in critical care. The expected end date is December 2006. More details can be found at www.icnarc.org/research/service-delivery/outreach.

[3] Guidelines for the development of outreach services have been published by the Intensive Care Society (ICS, 2002).

health care practitioners across all disciplines with the opportunity to gain the skills and knowledge to recognise the key signs of physiological deterioration, to initiate prompt treatment, and to readily obtain appropriate support from experienced colleagues.

According to the most recent reports on critical care services, the acquisition of the skills and knowledge identified above remains a key objective for acute hospitals and requires ongoing commitment and funding (DH and NHS Modernisation Agency, 2003; DH, 2005a). Significantly, this requirement for high dependency skills is now being mirrored in priorities for paediatric nursing (DH, 2001b), with considerable work ongoing throughout hospital trusts in the UK to produce a structured competency-based model for the provision of paediatric high dependency nursing care (Day *et al.*, 2005).

Critical care follow-up

Advances in support for patients recovering from critical illness have been another important output from the work of the critical care networks. The establishment of critical care follow-up clinics is a key initiative in enabling discharge and enhancing patients' experiences of critical care (Audit Commission, 1999; DH, 2001b). These clinics have evolved in both nurse-led (Glendenning, 2001; Cutler *et al.*, 2003) and doctor-led (Waldmann, 2002) formats. They have been instrumental in highlighting the vast array of significant problems experienced by critical care survivors (Jones *et al.*, 1998; Jones and Griffiths, 2000), which, if identified early in the recovery process, may help to prevent readmission and improve patients' quality of life. Nevertheless, a key issue with the continued development of follow-up clinics may be the inherent cost of such a service (Cutler *et al.*, 2003). However, although the anticipated costs may at first sight be considered untenable, it can be argued that they may be insignificant when compared with the daily cost of a critical care bed (Waldmann, 2002).

The Discovery Interview Process

A further initiative supporting the work of follow-up clinics has evolved from the directive to increase the involvement of patients and carers in improving services (DH, 2000a). Both as part of and separately from follow-up clinics, this has been enacted in critical care through the introduction of the Discovery Interview Process, which looks at patients' journeys through their whole health care experience and particularly through their experiences of critical care (NHS Modernisation Agency, 2004a). Whilst the need for further development in these processes has been acknowledged, early evaluation of Discovery Interviews has indicated their potential to lead to positive changes in care and to promote a culture that fosters patient involvement and patient-centred care (CHD Collaborative, 2005).

Care bundles for critical care

A more recent development in the Critical Care Programme has been the introduction of care bundles. Care bundles are a collection of evidence-based processes for patients undergoing a particular intervention, or with particular symptoms, which together have the potential to improve patient outcome (Fulbrook and Mooney, 2003). With an 'all or nothing' approach, all aspects must be completed to achieve optimum effectiveness. The strength of care bundles lies in the fact that they are a grouping of evidence-based practices. As emphasised by Fulbrook and Mooney (2003), it is anticipated that the effect of the whole will be greater than the sum of its parts. Care bundles have been in use in the United States for several years, and early evaluations related to ventilator care both there and in the UK are positive (Institute for Healthcare Improvement (IHI), 2005; NHS Modernisation Agency, 2005). However, whilst each element may have a well recognised evidence base, evidence in support of whole bundles is still very much in its infancy (IHI, 2005). Care bundles were introduced to the UK in 2002 and their development in critical care continues through established links with the critical care networks (ibid.). Care bundles that have been introduced in the UK include ventilator care, and related sedation protocols (Fulbrook and Mooney, 2003; NHS Modernisation Agency, 2005).

The review now turns to explore the issues that are particularly relevant for three specialist branches which make up critical care services: paediatric intensive care, emergency services and coronary care.

Challenges for specialist services within critical care

Challenges for paediatric nursing in critical care

The delivery of paediatric intensive care nursing (PIC) has experienced a period of change and development not unlike that in adult critical care. Two significant reports, *A Framework for the Future* (DH, 1997b) and *A Bridge to the Future* (DH, 1997c), focused on the provision, standards and nurse staffing requirements for the care of critically ill children. Levels of care were specified, and provided the basis for streamlining paediatric care across district general hospitals (DGHs) (level 1 and initiate level 2), lead centres (all levels plus support for DGHs), major acute hospitals (large throughput at all levels) and specialist hospitals (e.g. burns units) (DH, 1997b). Unfortunately, these levels of care are not directly comparable to those adopted later for adult critical care (thus causing potential for confusion), as level 2 care for children is likely to include intubation and possibly advanced respiratory support whereas level 2 care for adults does not (DH, 2000b).

In response, the focus for paediatric nursing has been on the development of an appropriately qualified workforce (i.e. a qualified children's nurse) to provide these levels of care, and, significantly, no matter what the location of care. However, implementing this has been fraught with difficulty as DGHs no longer offer nurses the same level of exposure to paediatric intensive care and thus they find it difficult to gain that initial experience and to maintain their skills (Camsooksai, 1999; Crabtree, 2001). As an alternative to these standards, Smith and Long (2002) suggest a framework that mimics the proposals laid down by the Royal College of Surgeons of England (RCSE, 2000, cited in Smith and Long, 2002). This framework matches training requirements to the level of service to be given, thus nurses required to care for level 1 patients would undertake a lower level of training than those required to care for children requiring level 3 care (Smith and Long, 2002). Whilst these authors acknowledge that this framework does not meet the standards as they are currently articulated by the Nursing and Midwifery Council, they argue that it provides opportunities for ensuring that all nurses working with children have the knowledge and skills to deliver paediatric care more safely to specified levels, with the support of an experienced practitioner (ibid.).

Reforms in emergency care services

The reforms proposed in the NHS Plan (DH, 2000a) also had far-reaching implications for the organisation and delivery of accident and emergency (A&E) services[4]. Challenging the increasingly poor experiences of patients, the NHS Plan set out a clear target to reduce waiting times for patients attending A&E. The Plan specified that, by the end of 2004, all patients should be discharged, admitted or transferred within 4 hours of arrival in the A&E department (ibid.). With these and other changes driven forward through a ten-year strategy, *Reforming Emergency Care* (DH, 2001c), and with considerable financial investment in the recruitment of A&E consultants and A&E nurses, by October 2004 progress towards this target was well advanced with over 96% of patients spending 4 hours or less in A&E (DH, 2004b). Reflecting the key thread running through all aspects of the NHS modernisation agenda, the strategy for A&E reform centred on the patient, their views and their experiences of the whole health care package. Working in partnership with both primary and secondary care providers, locally and across the country, collaboration and sharing of good practice such as that seen amongst critical care networks is evidenced in the modernisation of emergency services (ibid.). This collaboration and sense of partnership is seen at its best where the whole hospital and social services work together to manage bed allocations, admissions and discharges, with the clear aim of improving the patient's journey.

Nurses in A&E have been at the forefront of these achievements. In the care of minor injury patients, substantial rises in the number of emergency nurse practitioners have been central to the success of the 'See and Treat' initiative

---

[4] Increasingly, the term 'emergency' is being used as a substitute for the traditional term 'accident' and emergency', such as emergency nursing, emergency nurse or emergency department.

(DH, 2004b). Based on the principle that the first practitioner to see the patient is competent to assess, treat and discharge that patient, waiting times are kept to a minimum as each patient only requires a minimum time to treat (ibid.). Nurses are also playing a significant part in other developments in the emergency care arena, such as point of care testing; nurse prescribing; emergency care practitioner roles and minor injury units and walk-in centres (ibid.). These and other developments will be explored further in Chapter 6.

Critical care or coronary care?

As services have developed to provide a seamless and responsive experience for patients since the publication of the NHS Plan (DH, 2000a), so too have professional role boundaries been required to change in favour of delivering optimum patient care. A key example of this can be seen in the overlap between the roles of A&E and coronary care nurses.

Improvements in the diagnosis and treatment of patients suffering from coronary heart disease (CHD) have been driven forward following the publication of the White Paper, *Saving Lives: Our Healthier Nation* (DH, 1999a), followed soon afterwards by the *National Service Framework (NSF) for Coronary Heart Disease* (DH, 2000c). Recognising cardiovascular disease as the major cause of death in the UK among both men and women (DH, 1999a), this NSF is a 'blueprint for action' to reduce the incidence of CHD. The disparities and inequalities in cardiac care within the NHS in the late 1990s have been acknowledged, and this far-reaching NSF defines the type and standard of services to be provided, time frames for implementation, and guidance to reduce these inequalities. It has a pivotal target of reducing the death rate from CHD by at least 40% by 2010 (DH, 2000c).

Timely and appropriate administration of thrombolytic therapy is a key strand of this framework. With extensive research showing that thrombolytic treatment is most effective when given within the first 1–2 hours of the onset of the symptoms of myocardial infarction, the NSF sets a 60-minute target for call-to-needle times, i.e. the time lapsed from calling for help to administration of the thrombolysis, and a 20-minute target (reduced from 30 minutes in 2002) for door-to-needle times, so that patients are treated within 20 minutes of arriving at hospital (DH, 2004c; Smallwood, 2004).

Progress towards these targets has been significant. Over 80% of eligible patients were treated within 30 minutes of arrival at hospital in 2004 (DH, 2005b) compared with 38% reported in 2000 (DH, 2004c) and 54% treated within 60 minutes of calling for help, an increase from 24% (DH, 2005b). Nurses have played a key role in these accomplishments, with success emanating from the expansion of 'nurse-led thrombolysis' where nurses experienced in coronary care are responsible for the assessment and identification of patients requiring thrombolytic therapy, both in hospital (Quinn *et al.*, 1998; Rhodes and Quinn, 1999) and via telemedicine in conjunction with paramedic services (Cox, 2002). Nurse-initiated thrombolysis, where nurses assess the patient and administer thrombolytic therapy under patient group directives both in A&E

and CCU, is becoming increasingly well established with significant results (Heath *et al.*, 2003; Smallwood, 2004).

These achievements highlight the benefits of role expansion and working collaboratively, but these are not without risk and the less tangible implications for such developments will be explored further in Chapter 8. However, some of the most significant challenges for the NHS which are central to the provision of these enhanced services for patients relate to the NHS workforce. In the next section, the key challenges facing critical care nursing in this regard will be discussed.

Supporting and retaining the critical care workforce

Recruitment and retention of all staff within critical care is fundamental to the delivery of the modernisation agenda set out in the NHS Plan, particularly with respect to emergency care, elective surgery and the NHS Modernisation Agency Critical Care Programme. Despite a 33% increase in the number of nurses entering pre-registration courses (Nursing and Midwifery Council (NMC), 2001), and a reported gain of 67 503 more nurses employed in the NHS since 1997 (DH, 2004c), there continues to be evidence of nursing shortages, with vacancy rates of 3–10% across England (Buchanan *et al.*, 2002; DH, 2002b)[5]. Such vacancies can create problems as existing staff may experience a greater workload and a decrease in job satisfaction and morale, and ultimately may decide to leave. High levels of staff turnover and significant use of agency nurses serve to compound the problem (Buchanan *et al.*, 2002). It is also recognised that the nursing profession has an ageing workforce, with 24% of registered nurses reaching retirement age in the next few years (RCN, 2002). A report by the King's Fund in late 2002, *Great to be Grey*, warned that experienced and skilled NHS workers are retiring early due to the pressures of heavy workloads, long hours, lack of support and rigid career structures (Meadows, 2002). This suggests that the profession is at risk of losing a vast number of its most experienced workforce, and swiftly needs to invest in measures to retain existing staff and to prepare more junior nurses for the roles ahead of them.

The effects of nursing staff shortages are likely to be exacerbated by the changes in doctors' working hours and junior medical training arising from the European Working Time Directive (EWDT) (Council of the European Union, 1993) and the Modernising Medical Careers Programme (DH, 2004d) respectively. These developments will serve to improve working conditions for doctors by reducing the numbers of hours worked[6] and, as a result of a

---

[5] NHS Staff Vacancy Survey of all NHS trusts in England undertaken by Department of Health in 2002. A vacancy is defined as a funded post which the trust have actively been trying to fill but which has remained vacant for over 3 months (DH, 2002b).

[6] EWDT has had a phased introduction for trainee doctors, in which they must not exceed 56 hours/week by August 2007 and 48 hours by August 2009. Eleven hours of continuous rest must be provided in each 24-hour period (Academy of Medical Royal Colleges, 2004).

more comprehensive, contemporary training programme for junior doctors, should improve patient care (MMC, 2005). However, these developments will still create a gap in service that will need to be filled.

With regard to critical care nursing, staffing shortages may be more keenly felt as a result of increasing demands for the specific skills, knowledge and competencies characteristic of this group of professionals. Whilst the development and work of critical care outreach teams is to be applauded, this has been a drain on the specialist nursing staff resources positioned traditionally within critical care units[7]. This looks set to be exacerbated by the recruitment of critical care nurses to fill key roles within Hospital at Night Teams (Adam, 2004; NHS Modernisation Agency, 2004b). Moreover, role developments in areas of theatre practice, such as anaesthetic practitioners and advanced scrub practitioners/ first assistants, may serve, at least in the short term, to deplete the existing cadre of experienced theatre nurses and operating department practitioners (ODPs). This will only add to the pressures already experienced by this under-resourced workforce (Rollin, 2004; Turner and McLaughlan, 2005).

Recruitment and retention of staff were identified as key issues in the action plan for the modernisation of critical care (DH, 2001a), and their importance has been highlighted more recently in a specific Department of Health publication in June 2004 (DH, 2004e). This latter document identifies a range of case studies which reflect positive strategies for improving the recruitment and retention of all professional groups involved in critical care provision. Key factors which are considered to influence the success of such strategies include flexible and family-friendly working policies, opportunities for learning and professional/career development, feelings of being valued and respected, and experience of working in a good, supportive environment (Buchanan *et al.*, 2002; Finlayson, 2002; DH, 2004e).

Nurses in critical care have been shown to respond positively to responsibility, autonomy and new challenges (Coombs, 1991; Cartledge, 2001). It has been proposed that the provision of good supervision and opportunities for continuing professional development are considerable incentives to nurses looking to start or further their careers in critical care (Thomas, 1997; Cartledge, 2001). Indeed, as proposed by Ashworth (1996), it may be the very challenge of the ongoing professional development required to meet the changing and complex needs of critically ill patients that is a key factor in motivating nurses to remain within this speciality.

As indicated earlier in this chapter, critical care nurses have, perhaps more than other specialists, been at the forefront of job redesign and implementation of several initiatives (Table 3.3), many of which are strongly affiliated to *New Ways of Working* (DH, 2002c) and National Service Frameworks in critical care (DH, 2004c).

---

[7] Conversely, it has been proposed that outreach has the potential to increase recruitment to critical care because it has raised awareness of the critical care service (DH, 2004b).

Table 3.3 New ways of working in critical care.

Operating theatre practice	■ Anaesthetic practitioners ■ Advanced scrub practitioners/first assistants ■ Surgical care practitioners
Accident and emergency	■ Emergency nurse practitioners ■ Emergency care practitioners
Coronary care (often in conjunction with A&E)	■ Nurse-led thrombolysis ■ Nurse-initiated thrombolysis ■ Diagnostic telemedicine
Paediatric ICU	■ Paediatric outreach ■ Paediatric retrieval
Adult ICU	■ Critical care outreach practitioners ■ Hospital at Night Teams

Education for developing practice

The underlying ethos espoused by the Modernisation Agency for these developments reflects the intention that such innovation will allow practitioners to develop the breadth and depth of their practice, leading to enhanced job satisfaction, motivation and inspiration for staff, and ultimately result in the delivery of an improved range, standard and choice of services to patients and the retention of an effective and fulfilled workforce (DH, 2004a,e).

Central to the success of role development in any arena of practice is the provision of appropriate education and training. With the increasing acuity of patients in hospitals, pre-registration nursing programmes have been under pressure to ensure that nurses are 'fit for [the] purpose' of meeting the differing needs of patients in all care settings (DH, 1999b), with increased emphasis placed on gaining the high dependency skills and knowledge to care for level 1 patients. More recently, whilst extensive discussions focus on fitness for practice at point of registration, suggestions for a fifth branch of pre-registration nursing in acute/critical care to meet the needs of patients into the 21st century have been advocated (Scholes *et al.*, 2004).

In respect of post-registration education, emphasis has been placed on securing, through collaboration with higher education institutions (HEIs), a progressive programme of competency-based education that provides critical care nurses with the skills and knowledge appropriate to the patient group they will be required to care for (DH, 2001b). One of the challenges facing nurse managers, however, is whether they want such programmes to consolidate nurses' specialist skills acquired when starting out in critical care or to cultivate new ones (Scholes and Endacott, 2002). Reflecting on the situation in A&E nursing, it could be argued that the plethora of developing roles over the past few years has left this nursing speciality rather bereft of clear role boundaries and a career structure (Crouch and Jones, 1997), with an array of post-registration courses to choose from but no core standards to guide the skills and knowledge requirements for an A&E specialist nurse (Scholes and Endacott, 2002). This situation prompted the implementation of a feasibility study funded by the Royal College of Nursing (RCN) to explore the need for an emergency nursing faculty, with an integral competency framework for core and specific clinical competencies and a clear pathway for clinical career progression (Endacott *et al.*, 1999). This pilot study resulted in the RCN's endorsement of a Faculty of Emergency Nursing in 2003, and the Faculty are now in the final stages of refining their competencies, working in liaison with Skills for Health, the skills sector commissioned by the Department of Health to undertake specialist competency development work for the NHS (Skills for Health, 2003). For a full discussion on the impact of competency frameworks on clinical practice see Chapter 9.

Conclusion

In line with the time frames identified in *The Nursing Contribution* (DH, 2001a), the Modernisation Agency's Critical Care Programme came to a close at the end of 2004. However, it is anticipated that Strategic Health Authorities will take responsibility for the continued roll-out of the improvements already initiated (NHS Modernisation Agency, 2003b), and that they will be supported by the newly established NHS Institute for Learning, Skills and Innovation. Classified as being a 'Special Health Authority in England', the Institute's aim will be to provide ongoing support to the NHS and its workforce in taking forward the work started under the guise of the NHS Modernisation Agency (NHS Institute, 2005). For critical care, they will be supported through the National Critical Care Stakeholder Group which was formed in 2004 (McElligott, 2005).

The advances in service provision and the associated workforce issues discussed in this chapter have highlighted the pace of change prevalent in critical care nursing since 1999. These changes have much to commend them, not just for their potential to improve standards and experiences of care for patients, but also for the opportunities they may provide for employment and progression within the NHS for people who might previously have been or felt excluded, and for growing the NHS workforce (DH, 2004f). However, the increasing range of roles within the NHS, and in particular within critical care, should be greeted with some caution, particularly where existing patient care is at risk of becoming fragmented and task-, rather than person-centred. Moreover, the great number of trainees looking for supervision and support whilst undertaking work-based training and education has the potential to counter the benefits of these new roles and may further burden an overloaded workforce. In critical care settings, the demands for supervision are already at full stretch, with increasing numbers of pre-registration nursing students, operating department practitioner students, health care assistants, post-registration students, and, in the future, trainee doctors in their foundation years. Care must be taken to ensure that the needs of critically ill patients and their families are not jeopardised by these competing demands (Scholes, 2003).

The next section of the book turns to explore how practitioners can be facilitated throughout their career to achieve their potential and ultimately strive towards achieving expertise. The theoretical lens through which such facilitation is examined is that of role transition.

References

Academy of Medical Royal Colleges (2004) Implementing the European Working Time Directive. A position paper from the Academy of Medical Royal Colleges, London.
Adam S (2004) Plugging the gap – critical care skills are the current universal commodity. *Nursing in Critical Care* **9**(5): 195–198.
Ashworth P (1996) Editorial: Learning for life. *Intensive and Critical Care Nursing* **12**(1): 1.
Ashworth P (2000) Editorial: Nurse consultant – a role whose time has come. *Intensive and Critical Care Nursing* **16**(2): 61–62.
Atkinson BL (1994) Critical care today. In: Millar B and Burnard P (eds). *Critical Care Nursing: Caring for the Critically Ill Adult*. London: Baillière Tindall, pp. 3–19.
Audit Commission (1999) *Critical to Success: The Place of Efficient and Effective Critical Case Services within the Acute Hospital*. London: Audit Commission.
Ball C, Kirkby M & Williams S (2003) Effect of the critical care outreach team on patient survival to discharge from hospital and readmission to critical care: non-randomised population based study. *British Medical Journal* **327**(7422): 1014–1016.
Buchanan J, Finlayson B and Gough P (2002) *In Capital Health? Meeting the Challenges of London's Health Care Workforce*. London: King's Fund.
Camsooksai J (1999) The education needs of intensive care nurses caring for children in mainly adult units. *Nursing in Critical Care* **4**(4): 193–197.
Cartledge S (2001) Factors influencing the turnover of intensive care nurses. *Intensive and Critical Care Nursing* **17**(6): 348–355.
CHD Collaborative (2005) *Evaluation of Discovery Interviews: Final Report*. London: Matrix Research and Consultancy. Available at www.heart.nhs.uk/serviceimprovement/1338/4668/27794/Discovery%20Interviews%20final%20report%2025%20April.pdf (accessed 1 May 2005).
Coombs M (1991) Motivational strategies for intensive care nurses. *Intensive Care Nursing* **7**(2): 114–119.
Coombs M (1999) The challenge facing critical care nurses in the UK: a personal perspective. *Nursing in Critical Care* **4**(2): 81–84.
Coombs M and Dillon A (2002) Crossing boundaries, re-defining care: the role of the critical care outreach team. *Journal of Clinical Nursing* **11**: 387–393.
Council of the European Union (1993) *The organisation of working time (EC Directive 93/104/EC)*.
Cox H (2002) Transmission of a 12-lead electrocardiograph via telemedicine: a pilot study. *Nursing in Critical Care* **7**(1): 7–14.
Crabtree I (2001) 'A bridge to the future': impact on high dependency and intensive care. *Journal of Child Health Care* **5**(4): 150–154.
Crouch R and Jones G (1997) Towards a faculty of emergency nursing – planning for the future. *Emergency Nurse* **5**(6): 12–15.

Cutler L, Brightmore K, Colqhoun V, Dunstan J and Gay M (2003) Developing and evaluating critical care follow-up. *Nursing in Critical Care* **8**(3): 116–125.

Day H, Allen Z and Llewellyn L (2005) High dependency care: a model for development. *Paediatric Nursing* **17**(3): 24–28.

Department of Health (1992) *The Patient's Charter*. London: HMSO.

Department of Health (1997a) *The New NHS: Modern, Dependable*. London: HMSO.

Department of Health (1997b) *Paediatric Intensive Care 'A Framework for the Future'*. London: DH.

Department of Health (1997c) A Bridge to the Future. Nursing Standards, Education and Workforce Planning in Paediatric Intensive Care. Report of the Chief Nursing Officer's Taskforce. London: HMSO.

Department of Health (1999a) *Saving Lives: Our Healthier Nation*, popular summary. London: HMSO.

Department of Health (1999b) *Making a Difference: Strengthening the Nursing, Midwifery and Health Visiting Contribution to Health and Healthcare*. London: HMSO.

Department of Health (2000a) *The NHS Plan*. London: DH.

＊Department of Health (2000b) *Comprehensive Critical Care: A Review of Adult Critical Care Services*. London: DH.

Department of Health (2000c) *Coronary Heart Disease: National Service Framework for Coronary Heart Disease – Modern Standards and Service Models*. London: DH.

Department of Health (2000d) *Improving Working Lives Standard*. London: DH.

Department of Health (2001a) *The Nursing Contribution to the Provision of Comprehensive Critical Care for Adults: A Strategic Programme of Action*. London: DH.

Department of Health (2001b) *High Dependency Care for Children: Report of an Expert Advisory Group*. London: HMSO.

Department of Health (2001c) *Reforming Emergency Care – First Steps to a New Approach*. London: DH.

Department of Health (2002a) *Census Figures*. London: DH.

Department of Health (2002b) *NHS Staff Vacancy Survey 2002*. London: DH.

Department of Health (2002c) *Changing Workforce Programme: New Ways of Working in Health Care*. London: DH.

Department of Health (2004a) *The NHS Improvement Plan: Putting People at the Heart of Public Services*. London: DH.

Department of Health (2004b) *Transforming Emergency Care in England – A Report by Professor Sir George Alberti*. London: DH.

Department of Health (2004c) *The National Service Framework for Coronary Heart Disease: Winning the War on Heart Disease*. London: DH.

Department of Health (2004d) *Modernising Medical Careers: the Next Steps. The Future Shape of Foundation, Specialist and General Practice Training Programmes*. London: DH.

Department of Health (2004e) *The Recruitment and Retention of Staff in Critical Care*. London: DH.

Department of Health (2004f) *The NHS Knowledge and Skills Framework (NHS KSF) and the Development Review Process*. London: DH.

Department of Health (2004g) *Skills Escalator Resource Pack: Achieving Your Potential*. London: DH.

＊ Department of Health (2005a) *Quality Critical Care – Beyond 'Comprehensive Critical Care'*. London: DH.

Department of Health (2005b) *Coronary Heart Disease National Service Framework: Leading the Way – Progress Report 2005*. London: DH.

Department of Health and NHS Modernisation Agency (2003) *The National Outreach Report 2003*. London: NHS Modernisation Agency.

Endacott R, Edwards B, Crouch R, Castille K, Dolan B, Hamilton C, Jones G, MacPhee D, Manley K and Windle J (1999) Towards a faculty of emergency nursing. *Emergency Nurse* 7(5): 10–16.

Finlayson B (2002) *Counting the Smiles: Morale and Motivation in the NHS*. London: King's Fund.

Fulbrook P and Mooney S (2003) Care bundles in critical care: a practical approach to evidence-based practice. *Nursing in Critical Care* 8(6): 249–255.

Gibson JME (1997) Focus of nursing in critical and acute care settings: prevention or cure? *Intensive and Critical Care Nursing* 13: 163–166.

Glendenning A (2001) Intensive care follow-up: setting up a new practice area. *Nursing in Critical Care* 6(3): 128–132.

Heath SM, Bain RJI, Andrews A, Chida S, Kitchen SI and Walters MI (2003) Nurse initiated thrombolysis in the accident and emergency department: safe, accurate, and faster than fast track. *Emergency Medicine Journal* 20: 418–420.

Institute for Health Care Improvement (2005) *Bundle Up for Safety*. Available at www.ihi.org/IHI/Topics/Improvement/ImprovementMethods/ImprovementStories/BundleUpforSafety.htm (accessed 18 April 2005).

Intensive Care Society (2002) *Guidelines for the Introduction of Outreach Services*. London: ICS.

Jennett B (1990) Is intensive care worthwhile? *Care of the Critically Ill* 6(3): 85–88.

Jones C and Griffiths R (2000) Identifying post intensive care patients who may need physical rehabilitation. *Clinical Intensive Care* 11(1): 35–38.

Jones C, Humphris G and Griffiths R (1998) Psychological morbidity following critical illness – the rationale for care after intensive care. *Clinical Intensive Care* 9(5): 199–205.

King's Fund Centre (1989) Intensive care in the United Kingdom: report from the King's Fund panel. *Anaesthesia* 44: 428–431.

Leary T and Ridley S (2003) Impact of an outreach team on re-admissions to a critical care unit. *Anaesthesia* 58(4): 328–332.

McElligott M (2005) *Shaping the Future of Critical Care: The National Critical Care Stakeholders Group*. www.rcn.org.uk/members/yourspeciality/newsletter-plus/forum/news dated 26 January 2005 (accessed 6 April 2005).

McSherry R and Haddock J (1999) Evidence-based health care: its place within clinical governance. *British Journal of Nursing* 8(2): 113–117.

Meadows S (2002) *Great to be Grey: How Can the NHS Recruit and Retain More Older Staff?* London: King's Fund.

Modernising Medical Careers (2005) *New Training Programme Heralds a New Era in UK Medicine*. Available at www.mmc.nhs.uk/content.asp?ID=223&sector=news (accessed 4 May 2005).

NHS Institute (2005) *The NHS Institute for Learning, Skills and Innovation*. Accessible at http://www.institute.nhs.uk/.

NHS Modernisation Agency (2003a) *Achieving Real Improvement for the Benefit of Patients*. Annual Review 2002/2003. London: NHS Modernisation Agency.

NHS Modernisation Agency (2003b) *Commissioning Partnerships: The Contribution of Critical Care Networks*. London: NHS Modernisation Agency.

NHS Modernisation Agency (2004a) *A Guide for Using Discovery Interviews to Improve Care*. London: NHS Modernisation Agency.

NHS Modernisation Agency (2004b) *Hospital at Night*. www.modern.nhs.uk/hospitalatnight (accessed 30 April 2005).

NHS Modernisation Agency (2005) *10 High Impact Changes* (accessible through www.content.modern.nhs.uk/cmsWISE/HIC/HIC+Intro.htm

Nursing and Midwifery Council (NMC) (2001) *Nurse recruitment 'on target'*. NMC News 13 December 2001. www.nmc-uk.org (accessed 20 July 2002).

Pittard A (2003) Out of our reach? Assessing the impact of a critical care outreach service. *Anaesthesia* **58**(9): 882–885.

Quinn T, McDermott A and Caunt J (1998) Determining patients' suitability for thrombolysis: coronary care nurses' agreement with an expert cardiological 'gold standard' as assessed by clinical and electrocardiographic vignettes. *Intensive and Critical Care Nursing* **14**: 219–224.

Rhodes MA and Quinn T (1999) A pilot survey to investigate the nursing contribution to hospital-based patient assessment for thrombolysis in the West Midlands. *Clinical Effectiveness in Nursing* **3**: 53–74.

Rollin A-M (2004) Multidisciplinary working – the anaesthetic team. *British Journal of Anaesthetic and Recovery Nursing* **5**(3): 43–45.

Royal College of Nursing (2002) Nursing shortages will jeopardise NHS modernisation unless government delivers spending review, says RCN. RCN Online Press Archive 19 February 2002. www.rcn.org.uk/news/2002 (accessed 13 August 2002).

Royal College of Surgeons of England (2000) *Children's Surgery – A First Class Service*, cited in Smith J and Long T (2002) Confusing rhetoric with reality: achieving a balanced skill mix of nurses working with children. *Journal of Advanced Nursing* **40**(3): 258–266.

Scholes J (2003) The skills escalator: implications for critical care nursing. *Nursing in Critical Care* **8**(3): 93–95.

Scholes J and Endacott R (2002) *Evaluation of the Effectiveness of Educational Preparation for Critical Care Nursing*. London: English National Board for Nursing, Midwifery and Health Visiting.

Scholes J, Freeman F, Gray M, Wallis B, Robinson D, Matthews-Smith G and Miller C (2004) *Evaluation of Nurse Education Partnerships*. www.brighton.ac.uk/inam/research/projects/partnerships_report.pdf (accessed 13 April 2006).

Skills for Health (2003) *The Sector Skills Council for Health* (available at www.skillsforhealth.org.uk/).

Smallwood A (2004) Nurse-initiated thrombolysis: a systematic review of the literature. *Nursing in Critical Care* **9**(1): 4–12.

Smith G (2000) To M.E.T. or not to M.E.T. – that is the question. *Care of the Critically Ill* **16**, 198–199.

Smith J and Long T (2002) Confusing rhetoric with reality: achieving a balanced skill mix of nurses working with children. *Journal of Advanced Nursing* **40**(3): 258–266.

Smith G, Osgood V and Crane S (2002) ALERT – a multiprofessional training course in the care of the acutely ill adult patient. *Resuscitation* **52**(3): 281–286.

Thomas HS (1997) The lived experience of novice ICU nurses: a phenomenological study. Unpublished MSc Nursing Dissertation: RCN/University of Manchester.

Turner S and McLaughlan S (2005) An in-house course for first assistants (advanced scrub practitioners) in theatres. *British Journal of Perioperative Nursing* **15**(2): 57–60.

Waldmann C (2002) Setting up a doctor-led clinic. In Griffiths RD Jones C (eds). *Intensive Care Aftercare*. Oxford: Butterworth Heinemann.

Wigens L and Westwood S (2000) Issues surrounding educational preparation for intensive care nursing in the 21st century. *Intensive and Critical Care Nursing* **16**(4): 221–227.

Part 2
Facilitating learning transitions towards expertise in critical care nursing

Chapter 4
Role transition

Introduction

Having explored the context in which critical care practice is situated, this chapter sets out the theoretical framework through which individuals might be enabled to develop expertise and to progress in their careers. The literature on role transitions is divided into two broad areas, career and life event transitions, and these are introduced to put in context a model of learning transitions and how this might be harnessed to enable an individual to achieve their potential.

Theoretical perspective

Role transition refers to a situation where an individual changes from one set of expected positional behaviours in a social system to another (Allen and van de Vliert, 1984). All of us assume multiple social roles defined by age, occupation, family and social commitments. Throughout our private and public lives we continuously slough off one role and take on many others (Sokol and Louis, 1984). Role transition is therefore an integral phenomenon in our lives.

The exploration of role transition can broadly be divided into two key areas: life event and career transitions. Life event transitions significantly affect social status in the private sphere of people's lives, for example marriage, parenthood and bereavement (Moos and Schaeffer, 1986). Research in this area seeks to identify ways to facilitate individuals through the process of change, notably through counselling (Schlossberg, 1984).

The definition of a career transition is when one moves from one paid position to another (Nicholson and West, 1988). However, DiMarco (1997) extends the definition to include: 'a refocus or shifting of what you are doing with the work portion of your day' (ibid.: 1). Career transitions occur in the public sphere of people's lives and have traditionally been explored through the theoretical lens of occupational psychology. Research in this area focuses upon the movement into, out of and through occupational communities (Nicholson and West, 1988). However, increasingly it has become understood that primary transitions within either the public or private sphere of one's life can significantly impact upon the other, especially when the change strongly influences the behaviour and social identity of the transitioner (Allen and van de Vliert, 1984). When this happens it can be a major cause of stress (Schlossberg, 1984). In recognition of this, the contemporary literature tends to advocate a much more blended approach in facilitating occupational transitions. For example, life coaching with educational strategies helps foster leadership or managerial potential in the individual (Mellon and Sitkin, 2005).

Not all transitions are marked by crisis for the individual going through the change process although subtle changes to role can bring about significant behavioural change and alteration to self-identity (Allen and van de Vliert, 1984). Of note is the fact that the greater the change to self-identity the greater the associated emotional turmoil for the individual, especially if this is on the back of another transition from which the individual has not yet recovered (Williams, 2004). Importantly, we draw upon the experiences of past transitions to influence the way in which we cope with current change, and this can either ease or disrupt the process. Ultimately negative coping strategies may require intervention to enable the individual to adapt more positively to stressful life events or career transitions in the future (Fennell, 1999).

Role transition and nursing

We face many changes and challenges as we progress through our career from student nurse to expert practitioner. Revisiting the student role is a frequent phenomenon as we study for academic or clinical awards, or prepare to be a mentor, assessor, clinical supervisor, teacher or researcher. Most practitioners assume multiple roles with competing demands. Some roles may be overt, demonstrated by badge of office, uniform or conferment of a title. Others may be less obvious, yet nevertheless demand some form of adjustment or adaptation to fulfil the demands of that specific role.

Meleis (1994) places transition at the core of the discipline of nursing. She argues:

'Nursing is a discipline concerned with the process and experiences of human beings in transitions. It is also concerned with the development of nursing therapeutics to prevent, promote and deal with the experience and outcome of health transitions.'
(Meleis, 1994: 55)

Nursing research in this field has focused on transitions associated with life events, for example: how single adolescent girls transition into parenthood (Wuest, 1990); how poor relationships with partners and negative feelings about the physical changes associated with pregnancy influence the transition to motherhood (Flagler, 1990); how nurses handle the transition to care for the terminally ill in a hospice (Samarel, 1989); and how to facilitate the transition to woman for an elderly widow (Poncar, 1989). Other examples include the exploration of the transition to fatherhood and the impact this has on parenting skills (Parke, 1996; Holland, 1998; Jordan, 2005). In the sphere of primary care, interest has focused upon facilitating healthy transitions for asylum seekers (Johnson, 2003).

In critical care nursing the transitional model has been applied to help examine the experience of relatives and significant others as they adjust to the physical and emotional stress of a patient's admission to intensive care (Zainal and Scholes, 1997). Jones (2002) used life review as a therapeutic strategy to facilitate the recovery of young men following critical illness. In this instance, the process of recovery was conceptualised as a transitional process. As yet, this is a relatively untapped theoretical framework which could usefully be applied to expand our understanding of a number of transitions within critical care, for example, patients' and relatives' transitions when discharged from intensive to acute care settings; the examination of specific cultural needs of patients and relatives associated with new identities in a globalising society; and in the longer term the conditions and environments that promote and sustain healthy transitions from critical illness.

In the sphere of professional development, fully understanding career transitions from student to expert practitioner is important so that we may facilitate the individual to achieve their potential. Exploring the learning process in the development of expertise is the focus of this book. Fundamentally, I argue that to facilitate the transitions of others, be they patients in recovery, relatives of the critically ill, students or colleagues, one has to understand one's own experience of transition. This is not to suggest self-indulgent immersion in personal issues and the imposition of our experience on others, but to acknowledge these experiences so that we might foster empathic and compassionate strategies to nurture those experiencing a crisis through their change process. To do this we need to understand the elements which make up the transition process.

The process of role transition

Allen and van de Vliert (1984) define role transition as the point at which the individual has to move from one set of expected positional behaviours to another. They argue that this happens at a defined moment in time at the point at which someone (the focal person) assumes a new role. However, research into health care professionals in transition has suggested that this should be considered as a longitudinal process through which the individual has to adjust or adapt to the role expectations of the new position (Scholes, 1995). In the organisational psychology and management literature this is called 'transitioning', and lasts on average from 3 to 6 months (Mellon and Sitkin, 2005). Therefore, although a title may be conferred and outward vestiges of office may be on display on a given day, the process of assuming all the accepted behaviours of the new social role takes considerably longer.

In life event transitions, individuals may encounter a sudden event which affects their new role. Following the death of a spouse, a widow is immediately a widow. However, it takes far longer for her to make the transition through widowhood and find her new path in life (Poncar, 1989). Widowhood gives signals to the rest of society and with that role come certain privileges and obligations. For example, the widow is given permission to openly grieve, and society sets in place systems of support from either the family or the wider community. The expectation to wear black (or white in Asian societies) or withdraw from society is no longer the norm. It can, however, be a useful trigger to alert people to behave with sensitivity. This example also highlights the importance of role signals that alert people to a situation. This option is not available to all. In other significant life event transitions such as separation or divorce, the social roles do not command the same privileges and expectations of the widower or widow (Holmes and Rahe, 1967).[1] Indeed, it is only recently that the process of separation and divorce has been mooted as perhaps more stressful than widowhood, simply because society does not provide the same rights and obligations to the divorced person as are afforded to a widow or widower, and divorce can create additional financial and legal problems (Ball, 2003).

These two examples demonstrate 'role enactment' or role behaviour that validate the occupancy in any given social situation and give signs to others to help them respond in an appropriate way. How the individual enacts their social position will be affected by self-expectations and those of society. For example, McCoy (1996) argues that the negative effects of marital loss on depression are greater for people who believe in the permanence of marriage than those who do not. So this gives us the first element to examine: the circumstances and perceptions in which the individual finds themselves when confronting a transition, the phenomenon that Allen and van de Vliert (1984) describe as antecedent conditions (ibid.: 11).

Antecedent conditions

Antecedent conditions to a transition can be identified as either: chance events, societal forces, changes in role senders, change in capabilities or motives of the role sender, or change in capability and motives of the focal person (Allen and van de Vliert, 1984). This book mainly focuses upon the last category of

---

[1] The social readjustment scale (Holmes and Rahe, 1967) developed a life crisis scoring table. The highest score (100) was attributed to the death of a spouse, with divorce coming second scoring 73 and separation scoring 65. They posited that a series of experiences that scored over 150 would result in stress-related illness. Although the reliability of the original study was subsequently challenged (Krol and Schonfield, 1973), the scoring system is now considered in most health psychology training. Furthermore, reference is made to its use in many self-help web pages: a search engine hit 13 800 results in response to the search terms 'Holmes and Rahe' and 226 000 hits to the search terms 'life crisis scoring table' (14 January 2005).

Table 4.1 Antecedent conditions and examples in contemporary life.

Antecedent condition	Examples
Chance events	Winning the lottery Disaster Serious accident or illness Vacancy factor: relative staffing capacity
Societal forces	Government policy, priorities and provision Economy and employment Technological advances in health care
Changes in role senders	Service or resource reconfiguration Local policy application Career profiling and opportunities within workforce development planning Education commissioning strategies

Change in capabilities or motives of the role sender	Recruitment and retention initiatives
	Practice development initiatives
	Competency-based provision and education
	  opportunities
	Task and finish activities or specialist leadership
	  for certain aspects of practice within the unit

Change in capabilities or motives of the focal person	Personality characteristics and motivation Professional competence and profile Educational experiences Personal preferences, ambitions Work–life balance Personal responsibilities and roles

antecedent conditions. However, the others are worthy of mention as they might themselves become contextual factors that influence a nurse's transition to expertise. Table 4.1 sets out some examples in the context of health care and life experience.

The triggers for a role transition are often multifactorial. Rarely are they brought about by a single trigger. The vignette below illustrates how these theoretical concepts can be used to analyse a career transition for a critical care nurse.

Scenario 4.1: Factors that trigger a role transition into an outreach service

A member of the critical care outreach team has developed a serious illness that has resulted in her being put on long-term sick leave (chance event). Government policy, driving the need for acute care services to fit the concept of 'critical care without walls' (DH, 2000), has set the provision of critical care outreach services as a priority (societal force). The service in the local Trust has been established for 18 months, and is led by a nurse consultant. The Trust plans to expand the service to 24-hour cover (change in role senders) so they might fulfil the requirements of the Hospitals at Night service (change in societal forces). The Trust has fostered a policy that, in periods of long-term absence from work, health care practitioners, with appropriate competencies, can be seconded into other parts of the service as part of the continuing professional development programme. They have funding to back-fill the secondee's vacated post (change in capabilities or motives of the role senders). The applicant, a nurse with 5 years' experience of critical care practice, is seeking to expand her repertoire of experience through working as a member of the outreach team (change in the motives of the focal person). The applicant recognises that she will need a period of supervised practice with an experienced outreach practitioner to facilitate the application of knowledge to the new context of working within the outreach service (seeking to expand the range of capabilities of the focal person). This individual recognises this as an excellent opportunity to enhance her competencies and gain experience of outreach practice so that she might apply for a substantive post once the Trust implements their Hospitals at Night service (personal motivation and ambition).

It is important to analyse the antecedent conditions that trigger a role transition as they:

- fundamentally influence the individual's expectations of the role that they are about to assume; and
- make explicit how other role senders involved should act towards them.

This helps to determine if the expectations are realistic, understated or exaggerated.

In the example presented above, it might well be that the outreach team is seeking to develop new practitioners within the service, or, because of the profile of the team, is seeking a practitioner who has experience of providing the service. Without clarifying this most obvious issue (and because it seems so apparent it may go unstated), and taking account of other contextual factors, the level of support provided for the transitioner may be less than is required. In summary, to facilitate an effective transition, establishing realistic goals is clearly a very important part of the process. Critical to understanding someone's expectations is identifying the primary factors that triggered the transition in the first instance.

Expectations

Establishing the amount of difference in expected behaviours is essential. In recent years, job descriptions and competencies associated with any role have been widely introduced (DH, 2000, 2004). Although extremely useful in determining goals, this does not necessarily cover some implicit elements of role performance which are normatively governed (cohort defined), or determined locally through custom and practice. These aspects are usually learnt by socialisation into the role. Two examples where this is most acute are: for *novices* to the world of critical care nursing; or for experienced critical care nurses transferring to new units, whereby they become *newcomers* who have to learn the subcultural norms of the unit and adapt to subtle differences in the use of protocols or equipment. This experience may have the effect of temporarily rendering past experience redundant, until the focal person feels confident in assimilating or adapting past knowhow into their new role (Scholes and Smith, 1997).

New role expectations will be used as an evaluative standard for past performance and this can ultimately influence the focal person's confidence in their capacity to achieve the stated goals or role behaviours. Therefore, the meaning of the new role is greatly influenced by the one that preceded it. Furthermore, strategies to cope with the transitioning process are drawn from past experiences of managing change, be that personal or professional. In extreme cases this can result in a complete collapse in self-belief and a lack of confidence to perform even simple tasks. Conversely, this can result in an over-confident performance, assuming far too much or overstepping boundaries. This causes considerable alarm to role senders, especially if it is suspected that these actions are undertaken through unconscious incompetence (Scholes and Smith, 1997). Therefore, although the introduction of clear goals for the new post-holder are to be applauded in helping to clarify role expectations, the personal and professional background of the focal person will make this a unique experience and even skilled facilitators may be confounded by the lack of uniformity of response. This is obviously welcomed where roles require high levels of individuality and creativity, but may be less welcome for new post-holders in positions that make up the bulk of the workforce. Primarily these roles are standardised, and post-holders are required to contribute almost immediately to service provision (DH, 1999; UKCC, 1999). In these instances, self-doubt and anxiety that inhibit the assumption of role responsibilities are less well tolerated, especially if these exceed the 'normal' adaptive period (Kite, 1998; Scholes and Endacott, 2002).

The amount of time the individual has to anticipate the transition will affect preparation for the new role. The more an individual can control the transition, the better the anticipation of it (Allen and van de Vliert, 1984). Also, the more time the focal person can spend in a transitional, or in-between, position, the greater the anticipatory socialisation for the new role (Merton, 1957). In these positions, such as a period of supernumerary or supervised practice in formal preceptorship programmes, there are different privileges and obligations, which themselves can require role change and adaptive learning. The privileges are high levels of support and challenge, but the obligation on the focal person is to use that time well to help them adapt to the new demands of that role. In this situation, failure to use the time to address shortfalls in competence or adapt former know-how to the new situation might result in negative evaluations of performance that ultimately call into question the motivation of the transitioner (Scholes and Smith, 1997). Overly optimistic or pessimistic anticipation of what can be achieved in this period can result in additional strain (Allen and van de Vliert, 1984).

The focal person's past experience of high challenge and high support from mentors will ultimately influence their anticipation of as well as their reaction to these interventions. For example, many students who participated in the evaluation of the new Making a Difference curriculum expressed alarm at being directly questioned about their knowledge base (Scholes et al., 2004a). Furthermore, it was evident that students undertaking post-registration critical care courses equally found the high level of probing questions to which they were exposed in critical care settings, both before and after they were on the course, to be a new experience (Scholes and Endacott, 2002). This suggests that pre-registration students are not routinely challenged by their mentors (Scholes et al., 2004a). Furthermore, if students are not routinely receiving role models who question knowledge and directly observe performance to assure competence, the validity and reliability of the practice assessment process is in question (ENB/DH, 2001: 14). Perhaps more profoundly concerning is that these students are not learning how to question and support others. Thereby successive generations of students are exposed to an ever more diluted form of critical and supportive mentorship (Scholes et al., 2004b). However, students noticed that in certain clinical learning environments direct questioning was more apparent, for example in critical care and primary care settings. It is not coincidental that these environments are inhabited by practitioners who have undertaken specialist post-registration programmes. Furthermore, the nature of the specialities has resulted in practice educators specifically appointed to assess the competence of students on these programmes and enhance the knowledge base of the qualified teams in that locality or unit. They are therefore more likely to have been exposed to role models who have provided high challenge and high support. This experience helps to socialise successive generations of practitioners to do the same.

The examples provided so far have been ones whereby an individual has had some time to anticipate, prepare and hopefully experience a period of facilitated anticipatory socialisation into the new role. These individuals might have experienced a collective rite of passage (Glaser and Strauss, 1971; Boyanowsky, 1984), for example the graduation ceremony at the end of their training. However, although this marks the successful completion of their course and entry to the professional register, it does little to prepare the practitioner for the real-world experience of taking up their first qualified nurse post. The Vice Chancellor may well make the valedictory speech which includes the compulsory reference to 'now the real learning begins', but the event is more a celebration of success and closure to pre-registration student life than an awakening to a new, qualified, professional era. Transitioning takes place in the first few months of taking up the qualified role and this is why it is so important for the individual to have a preceptor to facilitate them through this period.

Role adjustment and role adaptation

The extent to which expectations are either confirmed or contradicted affects the outcome of the transition process. It has already been identified that unrealistic expectations, whether overly pessimistic or optimistic, can increase the amount of emotional stress for the transitioner and indeed their facilitators. However, an additional phenomenon needs to be considered and that is the impact of *contradiction* of expectations. If this occurs, the transitioner has to revisit, reconstruct, reframe and review perspectives to make sense of the experience. Although contradiction can increase the stress of the experience, it is core to experiential learning (Eraut, 1994). Therefore, helping an individual to expect contradiction and offering support through the experience can help to enhance experiential learning: a life skill essential for the transition to expertise.

A facilitated process of reflection is critical to enable the transitioner to learn meaningfully from such an encounter (Mezirow and Associates, 1990). Some suggest that reflection is a naturally occurring phenomenon and we all possess the skills with which to reflect if awakened from the latent state (Boyd and Fales, 1983). Boud *et al.* (1985: 3) view reflection as: 'a generic term for the intellectual activities in which individuals engage to explore their experiences to lead to new understanding and appreciations'. Schlossberg (1981: 5), however, argued that 'to change assumptions about oneself requires a corresponding change in one's behaviour and relationships'. Therefore, when a transitioner's expectations are contradicted, this will require significant *role adaptation* to accommodate the newly constructed perspectives and expected role behaviours. This has the potential to create considerable emotional stress, especially if this profoundly alters the self-identity of the transitioner. Conversely, when a transitioner has their expectations *confirmed*, this requires minimal *adjustment* and is far less stressful, emotional and demanding. This may be a good or bad thing depending on the stage at which the transitioner is met with confirmation and on whether, as a result, the individual then strives to avoid contradiction.

The premise on which this book is founded is that: reflection is inextricably linked to role transitions; role transitions are inextricably linked with contradictions; and contradiction is core to experiential learning. When experiential learning is reflected upon, the cycle starts again. Throughout this process, points of contradiction might trigger the individual to undertake formal learning. New learning takes time to embed into practice, but with purposive reflection the individual can recognise the transition effected by that learning encounter and progress in their quest for expertise.

However, without reflection and reconstructing expectations as a result of a new role, an individual may assume the title but fail to make the transition necessary to change behaviour and mind set to fit them for that role. The focal person might initially attempt to defend themselves from contradictory encounters, but this is time limited because it is too exhausting to be sustained.

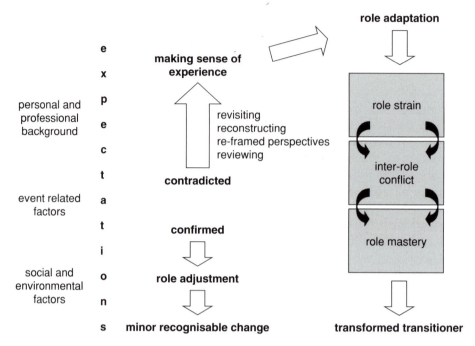

Fig. 4.1 Mapping the transitioner's experience.

In the meantime the focal person might superficially act out role behaviours, but to sustain this façade can generate role strain that ultimately leads to contradiction. However, *after* role adaptation, when the focal person finds that their goals set for that post are confirmed, this is a positive feedback loop. Successful transitioners are awakened to the fact that they will encounter contradictions from which they can learn in their everyday practice. Here we see that the transitioner embeds contradiction as an expectation into their changed landscape and thus the processes of change and learning are inextricably intertwined (Pollack and Brown, 1997). Figure 4.1 maps out the key elements of the transitioner's experience.

Role strain

The process of role transition can therefore lead to a variety of outcomes ranging from minimal disruption to the individual's psychological functioning to extreme stress and even emotional distress. But it should not be assumed that it will always lead to psychic turmoil (Glaser and Strauss, 1971). If the transition represents upward mobility or movement towards a desirable position that is anticipated with pleasure, and where the transition goals are clearly identified and there are unambiguous role expectations and support from role senders, the experience of role transition can be a positive one, especially if the roles have little importance to the focal person's social identity (Allen and van de Vliert, 1984). However, it is far more common for there to be some, if not a lot of, strain associated with role transition even under optimal conditions or when the shift is considered desirable. This is because the process of reflection, adaptation of behaviour and reconstruction of the self associated with the change demands a shift in the status quo. This can lead to anxiety, perplexity, disequilibrium and discomfort (ibid.).

Moderators

The amount of strain experienced by the transitioner is affected by factors known as moderators. These can exert influence at any stage along the process and sometimes exert influence at a number of points in the process. Some of the most influential moderators arise from the focal person's personality, for example, attributional style (locus of control), self-esteem or confidence, cognitive structure, social identity and level of arousability. Moderators that arise from an individual's social network include: one's social support system, and centrality of the role to self. Therefore, someone with high self-confidence, a high threshold to stress (level of arousability), and strong social support will have a different experience from someone with a different profile even though the two may undergo a similar transitional event (Allen and van de Vliert, 1984).

This is an important issue, as much of the literature on career transitions, and the literature on facilitating transitions to managerial and leadership positions, tends to be based on upwardly mobile, high achievers. Such individuals typically demonstrate a profile of high self-esteem, tolerance for high levels of risk and a high threshold against the adverse physiological effects of stress. However, nurses as a group tend to express low self-esteem, feel undervalued and may experience chronic fatigue as they struggle against the pressures of their working lives (Norris, 2000). This suggests that transitions throughout the nursing career need specific attention. The book is dedicated to enabling these transitioners to effectively achieve a more positive outcome.

Reactions

The response to strain brings about a number of reactions. These can be affective, and expressed as emotional responses such as depression, anxiety and anger. At a cognitive level, reactions can include, reflection, distraction or re-interpretation of events. The response can also be behavioural, either by taking action to regain control of the situation, or by engaging in acts that might reduce the strain: for example taking physical exercise, stimulants, night sedation, drugs or alcohol. Alternatively strategies to reduce the impact of the strain might be meditation, searching for information or undertaking new learning, or seeking the guidance of a mentor to help them make sense of the process.

In these examples it can be seen that some reactions are directed towards the self, and others are aimed at controlling the environment. Yet others are aimed at the moderators to help alter the self-concept (hence the wealth of available self-help literature to be found on the web), or at reinterpreting antecedent conditions or causal factors. Several of these strategies can be used at any one time and can be directed at more than one phase of the role transition process.

Consequences

This refers to the long-term impact on the psychological and physical health of the individual undergoing the transition. As Holmes and Rahe (1967) have depicted in their scoring system, the experience of multiple significant life-event or career transitions can have a serious effect on health. Likewise, the strategies used to reduce the impact of the strain can have longer term benefits (taking up an exercise programme and taking stress-relieving medication) or be detrimental to the health of the focal person (addictive properties of drugs, alcohol, chocolate, cola drinks, etc.). Moderators of and reactions to role transitions, and their consequences, are summarised in Fig. 4.2.

The psychological and objective beginnings of a transition do not necessarily coincide. In some instances this can be delayed; in others the psychological processes can proceed faster than the objective experience of transition. This can have one of two effects: the transitioner can have acquired the skills and have undergone changes to self and professional identity long before official recognition of the transition (Allen and van de Vliert, 1984). However, the converse is more often the norm, especially when the transition is affected by an educational experience, with alumnae taking up to two years to manifest signs of graduateness (Norris, 2000).

The emotional component of learning transitions is an under-researched area. However, interaction with students and career transitioners teaches us that the emotion associated with learning is a significant phenomenon. I will

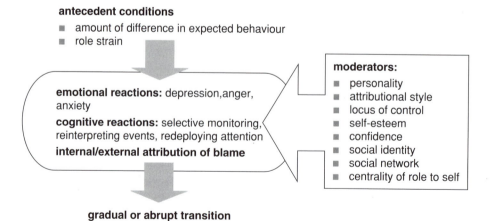

Fig. 4.2 Factors that can influence coping with life event transitions (adapted from Allen and van de Vliert, 1984).

use the case example of a group of Enrolled Nurses converting to Registered General Nurse[2] to explain some of the factors that can cause such strong emotional reactions. Although this study focuses upon one programme of study, the transitional phenomenon identified by this research can be used to help in understanding the processes other students encounter when exposed to formal or work-based learning experiences.

Career transitions: the impact on professional and personal identity

In a study of students undertaking a 12-month full-time course converting from Enrolled Nurse to Registered General Nurse, it was found that exposure to new knowledge, alongside assuming the role of student through which they could apply their new knowledge to practice, created a very significant transition that impacted on all aspects of the students' lives. In short, the process of reflecting on what they thought they knew in the light of new knowledge caused them to challenge a number of taken-for-granted assumptions in their personal and professional lives (Scholes, 1995). Hence, as they moved through the programme and as they reconstructed their perspective on practice and the profession, this fundamentally impacted upon how they reconstructed their personal identity (ibid.). As Allen and van de Vliert (1984) point out, the greater the impact on personal identity that any role transition might have, the greater the emotional experience and potential stress associated with the change process. Indeed, as these transitioners went through the course they described moving into new social arenas, forming new social networks and also changing their personal styling. Each one of these behavioural changes was an expression of the internal, intellectual and professional transition they had made. Most importantly, as they redefined themselves professionally, they also redefined themselves within existing relationships. Where partners or friends resented or tried to inhibit the process of change, the relationship itself could become threatened. The strain any educational programme places on relationships is a recognised phenomenon (Delamont *et al.*, 1997), but on this programme it seemed to be particularly high. Why should this be the case?

---

[2] The study recruited students undertaking an EN–RGN conversion course in five distinct programmes. Each programme was constructed as a 'case', subject to constant comparative analysis. Three courses ran the 12-month full-time programme leading to certification and RN qualification, a fourth led to a diploma and RN registration, and the final sample of students were undertaking the distance learning conversion programme run by the Open University. In total 12 students from each cohort or programme (case) took part in the longitudinal study to examine their experience of role transition on each of these programmes. Data were collected by an interview, called the reflective dialogue (Scholes and Freeman, 1994), observation and review of course documentation within the illuminative evaluation tradition (Parlett and Hamilton, 1972).

Re-writing the self

For many of the enrolled nurses who took part in the study, the role of second level nurse was stigmatic (Scholes, 1995). They had entered nursing with low self-esteem and doubt in their intellectual ability. Indeed for many this forecast of their capability had been set by poor results at school or cast-away comments by teachers that scarred the individual and made them live out a self-fulfilling prophecy of low attainment. In some cases, the students revealed a history of abuse which conferred in their minds a state of unworthiness.

When examining the role transition they went through, one of the greatest and most shocking challenges for the students to cope with was the experience of success. This demanded a re-writing of their life script from one of predictable failure or poor attainment to one of achievement. For them it was easier to believe in the negative, and a great deal of support and encouragement were needed to help them make the first tentative steps in redefining who they might become, to take joy in their success rather than see this as a step towards ultimate failure. As each assessment loomed, the fear would grow, starting perhaps with one individual that spread like a contagion through the group. As the results came out and they were rewarded with success, the fear would build to a climatic explosion of emotion, doubting the outcome and then eventually accepting that they had climbed another rung of the ladder, which potentially meant they had further to fall. It took an enormous leap of faith to recognise that they had the potential to keep moving forward, and to open up the possibilities and then take stock and celebrate their achievements. Success for the majority was a contradiction to their expectations and this ultimately affected how they viewed themselves.[3]

In this example, we can see how the construction of self is strongly aligned with the social identity of the transitioner and how this exacerbates the stress associated with the change process. These students were not simply undertaking a course of study: they were re-writing a life script that ascribed past negativity to history so they might embrace a positive although uncertain future. But because of this, and perhaps because of the condensed time frame (12 months) in which this process took place, the expression of their change manifested itself through alterations to personal styling and outward displays to people. They were changed: confident and more optimistic. In addition, as they learnt to recognise their potential and savour the success in their career, they felt less willing to accept social situations or relationships which intentionally kept them oppressed. With new knowledge came greater linguistic skills and critical abilities to challenge the status quo and assert themselves. With each small cycle of success and conferment of respect came optimism in the future

---

[3] This emotional roller coaster lasted throughout the course. I am aware of many of the original participants to that study, now eminent clinicians with a number of academic and professional attainments under their belt, who glow with the pride of having made that traumatic journey towards self-belief, yet who harbour a healthy acceptance of the need to keep on learning.

and growth in personal confidence. These people changed inside and out, and if the people close to them did not change with them, it gave rise to conflict.

Typologies of transition

It is interesting to note that some students, be they convertees, pre-registration students, or students on critical care pathways or taking research degrees, may show no signs of changing. Indeed, some educationalists, managers, mentors or colleagues might despair that they seem singularly untouched by the programme of study. Some might well have been sent on a programme in the hope that it would effect a gestaltic change in the individual. But, and this is important to note, individuals can defend themselves against such change, especially if they keep their personal identity separated from the transitional process. In this instance they superficially subscribe to a programme of study, defend themselves against situations whereby they might have to confront painful contradictions either to what they know or to how they see themselves in relation to new knowledge or their practice. Furthermore, by deliberately selecting a path of low challenge, by avoiding constructively critical assessment or exposure to new possibilities, they can acquire certificates but show no significant change to their professional or personal construction of self. These students can be described, using an ecological metaphor, as lobsters, migrating across the sea bed (or in this case through their careers) with a huge extended front claw grabbing at qualifications. But the lobster is a lobster: it does not change and if subjected to excessive pressure to effect a transition, it will withdraw and migrate to an environment where no such threats are to be found.

By far the greatest number of students could be described as developing transitioners, or continuing the ecological metaphor, as dragonflies. Here, in the early stage of development, the naiad lives on different foods from the adult form, the dragonfly. As they develop to the mature form they grow additional appendages (capabilities, competencies and academic awards) that enable flight (promotion and expanded roles) and bring the ability to eat different foods, thus ensuring they do not compete for food with the premature form, the naiad. This is most obviously demonstrated when a student revisits the same subject throughout their career adding more information to an established base, rather than re-examining the foundations upon which they have built this understanding. They can thus expand their understanding and manoeuvre with gradual growth into new roles. This approach requires less disruption for the student and indeed those around them, but it can generate such subtle change that outward signs of change seem less evident.

The third category are known as transformative transitioners. These are the people who had to confront radical contradiction, often through exposure to new knowledge that required them to reconstruct, redefine and review what they knew and what they did in former roles. These transitioners go through the most extreme emotional experience as they slough off their old role to take on the demands of the new one. For many, they may have to grieve for the certainty of the past role and learn a new way of being (or even re-write their life script, as described above) as an outcome. At this point they may seem to close down or retreat within themselves. This has been described as going through a 'black tunnel' during which time they are unable to explain to others how they are feeling, other than overwhelmed and in distress.

To return to the ecological metaphor, they are like a chrysalis transforming to a butterfly. The exterior appearance is one of quiescence, but inside the chrysalis the pupa's body is almost completely broken down and then reorganised (Buchsbaum, 1973: 321). This process is neither visible nor expected by the exterior appearance. During metamorphosis (chaos created by the redefinition of the past and reorganisation of the future), transformative transitioners are unable to make sense of the process and articulate that to others, and in the short term they can appear dysfunctional (or quiescent) to outsiders. When the metamorphosis is complete, the chrysalis (or protective cocoon of trust in the past) becomes constraining to the butterfly within. The butterfly has to break free of this constraint, and the chrysalis fractures along the lines of least resistance. New strategies for defence (insurance against threat) have been developed including: flight; compound eyes with colour vision; a pair of antennae; and sensory hairs (Buchsbaum, 1973: 315). Insurance against future threat for the transformative transitioner is the reshaped, reconstructed and redefined knowledge about nursing and future roles; and an increased sensitivity to the environment in which they are about to function (RGN). The chrysalis has served its purpose and the butterfly breaks free. After a brief refractory period, during which time the wings dry out (early weeks in the new role), the butterfly (focal person in new role) takes its first tentative flight (realisation of rehearsed role whilst a student or during a period of anticipatory socialisation), trusting in their reflexive management of the future.

Although this is the most radical form of transition and perhaps the one that causes the most immediate concern about them for role senders, the outcomes of transformation render the butterfly completely unrecognisable to the earlier form (past role). Furthermore, this is a one-way dynamic and significant role change that affects not only their professional identity but also their personal identity. This is but one example of how a career transition, facilitated by purposeful educational strategies, can, as a consequence, trigger other life-enhancing transitions.

The vicarious transitioner

This raises an important concept, the notion of a vicarious transitioner; someone in the slipstream of a transition who themselves has to make changes to fit in with the new social identity and behaviour of the primary transitioner. How many times have partners and friends had to unwittingly assume the role of vicarious transitioner as we progress through courses and assume new roles in practice, either through promotion or because of changes made to working practices? Indeed, to what extent have children had to make adjust-

Table 4.2 Summary of the types of transitions and their key characteristics (Scholes, 1995).

Model of conversion	Type of transition	Key characteristic
Awareness Developmental Transformative	Prospective Incremental Transformative	Compensatory – confirming Professional maturation Reflective – redefining
	Vicarious	Involuntary cascade effect

ments to accommodate their parent's part-time study or have partners had to adjust to the altered hours a new career demands? With each change has there been a trade-off which ultimately creates new demands, new roles and further transitions? To what extent has this led to explosive scenes, feelings of guilt and absolute promises of 'never again'?

The findings from this study indicate that a career transition cannot be viewed in isolation. Changes in career, especially those stimulated by an educational experience, have an impact on the personal identity of the transitioner. In these situations this can invariably trigger either minor or major life-event transitions. Therefore, when facilitating the transition of a colleague, one should consider the complex social and psychological upheaval this may create for them which can, in the short term, affect their performance at work. Furthermore, it suggests that, when facilitating others, focusing concern solely on the students who appear to be excessively stressed by their course can lead to less attention being paid to the students who appear apparently unphased by their situation. It is vital that these students be evaluated as well and offered facilitated and critical reflection to enable them to identify contradiction and make the most of their learning opportunities. A string of qualifications is meaningless if this has not ultimately affected the professional transition of the practitioner. For a summary of the types of transitions and their key characteristics, see Table 4.2.

In this chapter the process of role transition has been dissected into analytical segments. The purpose has been to provide a framework within which to assess one's own transition as well as that of others. In this way an individual learning plan can be negotiated between the transitioner and their facilitator to help the individual through their change process and help to explain why this can be such an emotionally challenging experience. The framework below sets out structural activities that form part of any learning plan.

Facilitating learning transitions in the induction period

The learning transition when taking up a new post or starting out in a new allocation can be divided into four key phases:

(1) **Preparation**, or activities undertaken prior to taking up a new post.
(2) **Encounter**, the first days in the new post.
(3) **Adjustment**, the transitioning period which can last up to 6 months.
(4) **Stabilisation**, a point of consolidation and role comfort whereby the transitioner has changed behaviour, attitude and identity to fit with the new role (Nicholson and West, 1988).

During these four phases the transitioner and their facilitator are urged to acknowledge, legitimate and where necessary address (through empathic and

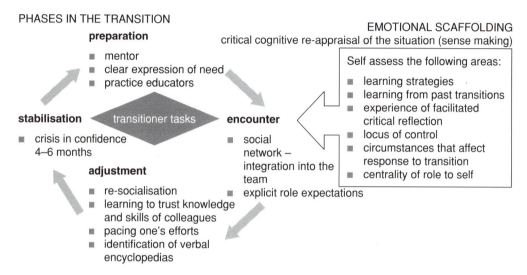

Fig. 4.3 Factors to consider for the transitioner.

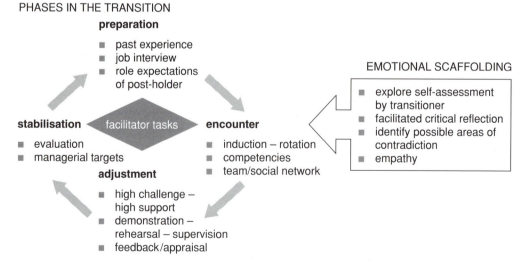

Fig. 4.4 Factors to consider for the facilitator.

facilitated cognitive reappraisal of events), the emotional components of such role change. In this way a facilitator is providing the emotional scaffolding to enable the transitioner to feel safe to address new learning that can alter both their behaviour and identity and truly fulfil the expectations of their new role. Figures 4.3 and 4.4 set out the factors that need to be considered by transitioners and their facilitators to help them maximise the learning potential of the experience.

The next chapter will explore the impact of formal education on the development of critical care practitioners on pre-registration and post-registration programmes, and will provide some detail of how to apply learning transition theory to practice.

References

Allen V and van de Vliert E (1984) *Role Transitions: Explorations and Explanations.* NATO Conference Series. Series III: Human Factors. New York: Plenum Press.

Ball M (2003) Which costs more, a wedding or divorce? http://money.msn.co.uk/planninglife_events/getting married/insight/weddedfinancialbliss (accessed 14 January 2005).

Boud D, Keogh R and Walker D (1985) *Reflection: Turning Experience into Learning.* London: Kogan Page.

Boyanowsky E (1984) Self-identity change and the role transition process. In Allen V and van de Vliert E (eds). *Role Transitions: Explorations and Explanations.* NATO Conference Series. Series III: Human Factors, New York: Plenum Press: pp. 39–52.

Boyd E and Fales A (1983) Reflective learning: key to learning from experience. *Journal of Humanistic Psychology* **23**(2): 99–117.

Buchsbaum R (1973) *Animals without Backbones: 2.* Harmondsworth: Penguin.

Delamont S, Atkinson P and Parry O (1997) *Supervising the PhD. A Guide to Success.* Buckingham: The Society of Research into Higher Education and Open University Press.

Department of Health (1999) *Making a Difference, Strengthening the Nursing, Midwifery and Health Visiting Contribution to Health and Healthcare.* London: DH.

Department of Health (2000) *Comprehensive Critical Care: A Review of Adult Critical Care Services.* London: DH.

Department of Health (2004) *The NHS Knowledge and Skills Framework (NHS KSF) and the Development Review Process.* London: DH.

DiMarco C (1997) *Career Transitions: A Journey of Survival and Growth.* Scottsdale, Arizona: Gorsuch Scarisbrick.

English National Board/Department of Health (2001) *Placements in Focus. Guidance in Practice for Health Care Professionals.* London: ENB/DH.

Eraut M (1994) *Developing Professional Knowledge and Competence.* London: Falmer Press.

Fennell M (1999) *Overcoming Low Self-esteem: A Self-help Guide Using Cognitive Behavioural Techniques.* London: Robinson.

Flagler S (1990) Relationships between stated feelings and measures of maternal adjustment. *Journal of Obstetric, Gynaecologic and Neonatal Nursing* **19**(5): 411–416.

Glaser B and Strauss A (1971) *Status Passage.* Chicago: Aldine.

Holland A (1998) Changing families, challenging futures. *6th Australian Institute of Family Studies Conference*, Melbourne, 25–27 November. http://aifs.gov.au/institute/afrc6papers/holland.html (accessed 15 January 2005).

Holmes T and Rahe R (1967) Social Readjustment Scale. Available from: http://www.mindtools.com/smlcu.html (accessed 15 January 2005).

Johnson M (2003) Asylum seekers in dispersal – health care issues. Home Office Online report 13 March 2003: publications.rds@homeoffice.gsi.gov.uk (accessed 15 January 2005).

Jones C (2002) Life review following critical illness in young men. Unpublished PhD Thesis, Liverpool Sir John Moores University.

Jordan W (2005) Role transitions: a review of the Literature. National Centre on Fathers and Families (NCOFF). Brief http://www.ncoff.gse.upenn.edu (accessed 15 January 2005).

Kite K (1998) Learning to doubt: the professional development of nurses in one intensive therapy unit. Unpublished PhD Thesis, University of East Anglia.

Krol W and Schonfield J (1973) Letter: Reliability study of the Holmes and Rahe Schedule of Recent Experiences. *Psychosomatic Medicine* **35**(5): 436–439.

McCoy J (1996) *Divorce Matters. Coping with Stress and Change*. Ames, Iowa: Iowa State University.

Meleis A (1994) A commitment to making a difference: nursing care and research for the future. Working Group of European Nurse Researchers (WENR) The Contribution of Nursing Research: past, present and future. Proceedings, Vol 1: 7th Biennial Conference, Oslo, Norway 3–6 July. Oslo: Falch Hurtigtrykk, pp. 47–56.

Mellon E and Sitkin S (2005) Managerial Transitions. Duke Corporation Education Strategy Execution through education. www.dukece.com/pdf/managerialtransitions (accessed 14 January 2005).

Merton R (1957) *Social Theory and Social Structure*. Glencoe, Ill: Free Press.

Mezirow J and Associates (1990) *Fostering Critical Reflection in Adulthood. A Guide to Transformative and Emancipatory Learning*. San Francisco, CA: Jossey Bass.

Moos R and Schaeffer J (1986) *Coping with Life Crises. An Integrated Approach*. New York: Plenum Press.

Nicholson N and West M (1988) *Managerial Job Change: Men and Women in Transition*. Cambridge: Cambridge University Press.

Norris M (2000) Contextual factors that enable or disable nurses' professional practice. Unpublished DPhil Thesis, University of Sussex.

Parlett M and Hamilton D (1972) Evaluation as illumination: a new approach to the study of innovatory programmes. Occasional Paper 9. Centre for Research in Educational Sciences, Edinburgh, and reproduced in Murphy R and Torrance H (1987) (eds). *Evaluating Education: Issues and Methods*. London: Paul Chapman Publishing.

Parke R (1996) *Fatherhood*. Cambridge: Harvard University Press.

Pollack M and Brown K (1997) *Learning and Transitions in the Careers of Librarians*. International Federation of Library Associations 63rd General Conference, Copenhagen. www.ifla.org/IV/ifla63/63alpha.htm (accessed 15 January 2005).

Poncar P (1989) The elderly widow: easing her role transition from widow to woman. *Journal of Psychosocial and Mental Health Services* **2**: 6–8, 10–11, 39–40.

Samarel N (1989) Caring for the living and dying: a study of role transitions. *International Journal of Nursing Studies* **26**(4): 313–326.

Schlossberg N (1981) A model for analyzing human adaptation to transition. *Counselling Psychologist* **9**(2): 2–18.

Schlossberg N (1984) *Counselling Adults in Transition: Linking Practice with Theory*. New York: Springer.

Scholes J (1995) An exploration of role transition in students converting from Enrolled Nurse (General) to Registered General Nurses (Unpublished DPhil, Sussex University).

Scholes J and Endacott R (2002) Evaluation of the effectiveness of educational preparation for critical care nursing. *ENB Research Highlights* **49**: 1–6.

Scholes J and Freeman M (1994) The reflective dialogue and repertory grid: a research approach to identify the unique therapeutic contribution of nursing, midwifery or health visiting to the therapeutic milieu. *Journal of Advanced Nursing* **20**: 885–893.

Scholes J. and Smith M (1997) *Starting Afresh: the Impact of the Critical Care Milieu on Newcomers and Novices*. ITU NDU Occasional Paper Series Number 1 (University of Brighton) [ISBN 1 87 196692 2].

Scholes J, Freeman M, Gray M, Wallis B, Robinson D, Matthews Smith G and Miller C (2004a) Evaluation of nurse education partnership. www.brighton.ac.uk/inam/ research/projects/partnerships_report.pdf (accessed 15 January 2005).

Scholes J, Webb C, Gray M, Endacott R, Miller C, Jasper M and McMullan M (2004b) Making portfolios work in practice. *Journal of Advanced Nursing* **46**(6): 595–603.

Sokol M and Louis M (1984) Career transitions and life event adaptation: integrating alternative perspectives on role transitions. In Allen V and van de Vliert E (eds). *Role Transitions: Explorations and Explanations*. NATO Conference Series. Series III: Human Factors. New York: Plenum Press, pp. 81–94.

UKCC (1999) *Fitness for Practice*. London: United Kingdom Central Council for Nursing, Midwifery and Health Visiting.

Williams D (2004) Life events and career change: transition psychology in practice. British Psychological Society's Occupational Psychology Conference, January 1999, updated 6 April 2004 www.eoslifework.co.uk/transprac.htm (accessed 15 January 2005).

Wuest J (1990) Trying it on for size: mutual support in role transition for pregnant teens and student nurses. *Health Care for Women International* **11**(4): 383–392.

Zainal G and Scholes J (1997) *Adapting to Crisis: the Relatives' Experience of Intensive care and the Nurse's Therapeutic Role with the Family*. ITU NDU Occasional Paper Series Number 3 (University of Brighton) [ISBN 1 87196674 4].

Chapter 5
Learning and transitions

Introduction

This chapter examines the various formal learning experiences that critical care nurses encounter and how these may impact on role transitions. I map educational provision from pre-registration preparation to post-registration specialist competency acquisition. This serves as a backdrop to inform the mentor as to how they can make a diagnosis of the student's learning needs and identify ways in which they can facilitate transition into critical care nursing using the models set out in Figs 4.3 and 4.4 (page 72). The chapter also addresses informal learning experiences that strongly influence the way in which critical care nurses acquire the necessary skills, knowledge and attitude for professional practice, notably the power of socialisation. It follows with a critical examination of the way in which the provision for formal education has changed and the potential consequence this might have for learning.

Pre-registration exposure to critical care nursing

When a student enters a critical care environment, it might be their first exposure to the subcultural world of that department. Some may have worked in this environment as a health care assistant (HCA), or experienced care first hand as a patient or as their relative, but for the majority this is their first encounter. With the introduction of the Project 2000 curriculum, fewer students were routinely allocated to critical care environments (Durston and Rance, 1995). Some were allocated to coronary care units, especially when this was attached to a medical ward, others went to accident and emergency or theatres, but fewer were allocated to intensive care settings unless as an elective (Kite, 1998). During the late 1980s and 1990s, allocations to the theatre department were discontinued in favour of a follow-through model, whereby the student was exposed to all the key events that made up the patient's surgical experience (Radford, 1998). The intention was to enable the student to identify with the holistic package of care rather than limit their experience to observing a series of surgical procedures. This became extremely unpopular with theatre nurses who feared this would have a devastating impact on recruitment to the department (Barker, 1996). Furthermore, offence was taken by theatre nurses because this implied that the value of nursing in that environment was in question (Jones, 1990; Conway, 1995; Willis, 1998).

Although theatres suffered the most explicit withdrawal of pre-registration students from the environment, other critical care environments saw a reduction in the number of students gaining valuable learning about care of the critically ill patient. This has inevitably had an impact on the skills and knowledge of newly qualified staff (Walker, 2001). Fundamentally, this has been one of the factors contributing to suboptimal ward care for rapidly deteriorating patients (McQuillan *et al.*, 1998).

The need for explicit critical care competencies or skills training within the pre-registration nursing programme was identified (DH, 1999, 2001). With the introduction of the new competency-based/Making a Difference/partnership curriculum (UKCC, 1999)[1], students were to undertake a placement in which they could learn the skills to care for the critically ill. The aim was to enable newly qualified nurses to recognise and respond to rapidly deteriorating patients (DH, 2001). The evaluation of the new partnership curriculum included an examination of what students learnt from an allocation to critical care to see if in any way these ambitions had been realised (Scholes *et al.*, 2004).

Making a difference? Student placements in critical care

One of the key issues for higher education institutions (HEIs) implementing the new curriculum was finding an adequate number of placements to provide a critical care experience for the expanded student numbers.[2] In response, many HEIs had to stretch the definition of a critical care or high dependency allocation to include environments caring for patients with 'complex needs'. However, in the main, students were allocated to environments such as theatres, anaesthetics and recovery, CCU, ITU or A&E.

---

[1] The curriculum has been called by all three names: 'Making a difference', as it was in response to the Government's report on the contribution of nursing and midwifery (DH, 1999), 'competency-based' curriculum in response to the Peach Report (UKCC, 1999), which identified the curriculum needs to be far more skills and competency based to enable the newly qualified staff to be 'fit for purpose'; and finally, the 'partnership curriculum' by the DH as they saw that the key way forward to redress this apparent need was through closer partnership between HEIs and Trusts to create more effective learning environments in practice as well as in the academic setting (Scholes *et al.*, 2004).

[2] One of the Government targets in the modernisation programme of the NHS was to increase the number of nurses in the NHS. One way was through increasing the number of student commissions. As an outcome, HEIs and Trusts had to rapidly expand the placement circuit to accommodate more students who were spending longer in practice throughout their pre-registration programme (Scholes *et al.*, 2004).

As part of the evaluation, a survey of students in the third year of their branch programme was undertaken. This would have reached the students in the last six months of their training.[3] Of the 370 adult student respondents, 36 stated that they had not had a critical care placement, although by far the majority ($n = 209$) had one placement; 77 claimed to have had two and 34 three. Although a placement had been distinguished from a 'visit', 14 students identified that they had between four and eight placements in a critical care, high dependency or complex needs environment during their branch programme (IES Survey, 2003). However, an analysis of the demonstration sites' curricula indicated that no single school had this number of placements in their branch programme, suggesting that these respondents had undertaken a sequence of visits or were on a circuit of experience and this formed their critical care placement.

Feedback from students indicated that the critical care placements were extremely popular, and they had a significant impact on consolidating knowledge (notably around biological science) and boosted students' confidence in being able to respond to the needs of sicker patients and/or emergencies (Scholes *et al.*, 2004).

The best features of a high dependency/complex needs/critical care environment were cited by students as:

- practical experience/patient contact/linking theory to practice;
- supportive staff;
- good learning environment/setting well managed;
- good assessor/mentor;
- team meetings/teamwork;
- variety of work;
- variety of patients.

---

[3] Accessing students by survey proved to be difficult. The aim had been to survey students in the Common Foundation Programme (CFP) and do a repeat survey in the final six months of their branch programme. The Data Protection Act prohibited HEIs from releasing details about the student cohort. Therefore, the researchers sent surveys to the HEI demonstration sites and requested that an administrator select every third student off their records and forward the survey to them. They were then asked to keep a copy of the labels so that, when the repeat survey was sent, the same students would receive a copy of the survey. Although this addressed the ethical and legal issue of access to student information, it proved to be a methodological challenge because the researchers had no control over when the surveys were sent and how many reached the students. On reflection it would have yielded a better response, and given the researchers greater confidence in the response rate to the survey, if these had been handed out in face-to-face contact with the student cohort whilst on visits to the HEI. In total 1462 surveys were sent to the HEIs. The first survey resulted in 760 being returned (548 from adult branch students and 201 from mental health students), but in the second survey this had dropped further to a response of 509 (370 adult branch student and 136 mental health students – 3 were unidentifed). As stated, this approach meant that the research team was unable to reliably state the response rate as we have no way of knowing how many actually reached their destination (IES Survey, 2003).

One of the most important issues for students (mental health and adult branch students) was the increased staff-to-patient ratio found on critical care and high dependency units, which also resulted in them being exposed to one-to-one supervision. This gave students the opportunity to ask questions, and to be involved in discussion about care and in debriefing after working with a patient. The students were encouraged to develop their fundamental nursing skills but also learn some new technical skills, for example measuring central venous pressure (CVP) or electrocardiac monitoring, and develop their understanding of other physiological recordings (e.g. the meaning of blood gas results). Some students reported that they were limited in the range of activities they could do even under supervision, but accepted this because of the highly technical nature of the placement. Students therefore valued these placements as they provided, in their terms, higher order learning opportunities which helped to: sharpen their understanding of the meaning of results; and provide experiences which furnished their need to cope with more technical equipment than they might see on the ward.

Students particularly enjoyed the approach to patient handover and report, which enabled them to slowly assimilate all the information about a patient. In ward handovers, where vast amounts of information were conveyed, the students found it hard to recognise the significance of all the issues raised and to prioritise the questions they should ask or the planning of the care for a group of patients. In critical care environments, students were exposed to staff questioning their colleagues and seeking clarification at handover, and this gave them confidence to foster a more questioning stance with their mentors.

In the survey, students rated good mentorship and support as two of the top three things about any placement (IES Survey, 2003). When asked about areas for improvement in a critical care placement, only 14% of the respondents identified more support and time with the mentor and 17% cited the need for better staff attitudes towards students (ibid.). These responses indicated that high dependency and critical care environments fared considerably better than other acute care areas. This was encouraging because the students identified that one of the key features that influenced their decision on career destination was staff attitude and support whilst they were on their placement as a student (Scholes *et al.*, 2004).

Outreach: learning critical care skills in the acute care environment

Within the orbit of the definition of critical care without walls, whereby: '. . . *each critically ill patient, wherever they are located in the hospital, should have skilled critical care nursing available either to care directly for them, or to advise on the care required to meet their needs*' (DH, 2000, paragraph 52), students could potentially acquire these skills from any acute care setting where such a service has been established (Coad *et al.*, 2002). However, to be effective, remedial work needed to be done with the qualified staff to ensure they had the appropriate skills to share with the pre-registration students (Plowright *et al.*, 2005).

A number of reports have highlighted inadequate or suboptimal ward care for the critically ill (e.g. Garrard and Young, 1998). McQuillan *et al.* (1998) identified that patients admitted to ICU were in an advanced stage of their illness and more timely and appropriate care might have prevented their admission in the first place. McGloin *et al.* (1999) estimated that two in five ICU admissions were due to inadequate ward care. Suboptimal ward care was linked with poor preparation and inadequate support and supervision of junior doctors and nurses (Audit Commission, 1999). In addition, the infrequent exposure to the critically sick on the wards meant that the staff had a reduced opportunity to develop competency in this aspect of care and to feel confident through consolidation or reflection because they had a number of other patients to care for at the same time (Carberry, 2002; Coad *et al.*, 2002; Odell *et al.*, 2002). Even when those skills were consolidated, the potential competency and knowledge pool was diluted by the rapid turnover of staff in the acute care wards (Odell *et al.*, 2002).

A number of studies undertaken by outreach teams illustrated that there remains the problem of identifying the critically sick and then acting in a timely fashion to ensure appropriate action is taken (Carberry, 2002; Coad *et al.*, 2002; Odell *et al.*, 2002; DH and NHS Modernisation Agency, 2003). Nurses might well have had a 'concern' for the patient, but found difficulty in expressing this in a language that would initiate appropriate action or review by a specialist team (Kenward and Hodgetts, 2002). To assist staff, early warning scores have been introduced whereby charts are marked to identify potential danger signs in the patient's breathing and circulation (Morgan *et al.*, 1997). This has proven to be a useful tool to alert staff to the imminent threat to the patient's condition (Stenhouse *et al.*, 2000), but there is no evidence of the tool's sensitivity and specificity (Goldhill *et al.*, 1999). To be used with any effect, education and support are critical (Coad *et al.*, 2002) to enable the nurse to undertake an initial assessment and report the findings with confidence and authority to outreach or patient at risk teams (Richardson *et al.*, 2004; Plowright *et al.*, 2005).

In response to this need, Trusts were urged to develop a coherent educational strategy in association with the workforce planners and HEIs, so that staff could meet the needs of the critically sick (DH and NHS Modernisation Agency, 2003). A variety of courses have been developed including advanced life support (ALS), advanced trauma life support, care of the critically ill surgical patient (CCriSP), and acute life-threatening events, recognition and treatment (ALERT). Each one uses a structured approach to assess priorities and manage the critically ill patient. The ALERT course has been one of the most extensive programmes used to develop skills among ward staff (Smith *et al.*, 2002).

This suggests that alongside the lack of experience of working with critically ill patients the nurses' knowledge base with which to identify the 'at risk factors' is weak (DH and NHS Modernisation Agency, 2003). For example, 80% of patients admitted to ITU had abnormal respiratory and heart rates and oxygen levels in the previous 24 hours which had not been acted upon until the patient 'collapsed' (Goldhill *et al.*, 1999). Chellel *et al.* (2002) identified that the respiratory rate frequently went unrecorded, and attributed this to the electronic recording of blood pressure and pulse, which prompted the nurse to record findings from the visual display and thereby omit observing the patient's respiratory pattern or palpating a pulse, which also gave the opportunity to feel for temperature, look at the patient's skin colour and texture and make an assessment of their consciousness level (Smith, 1988). In addition, inaccurate recordings of fluid intake and output meant that invaluable information about the patient's renal function went unnoticed (Chellel *et al.*, 2002; Wood *et al.*, 2004).

Learning the science to inform critical care skills

In many wards, the recording of physiological parameters has been delegated to HCAs. Students might well be asked to undertake these observations, but frequently did not acknowledge the critical elements of that assessment process, despite the number of times in one day they might be required to do this assessment (Scholes *et al.*, 2004). The denigration of such an activity as a routine or mundane task has obscured the professional judgement required to make sense of the information. In addition, the reduced emphasis on anatomy and physiology teaching within the curriculum has had a negative impact. A number of factors have been identified including: the reduction in hours spent addressing basic physiology; the chosen teaching method and when this pedagogy was addressed in the curriculum; and finally the lack of examples to apply the theory to clinical scenarios (ibid.). Furthermore, decades of poor quality physiology teaching and assessment have resulted in mentors with a weak knowledge base on which to judge the knowledge and skills of the students they assess (Akinsanya, 1985; Eraut *et al.*, 1995; Scholes *et al.*, 2004)[4]. Therefore, poor theoretical preparation and lack of clinical experience

---

[4] This problem is not isolated to ward staff and pre-registration students. Many D grade competence packages for critical care staff have invested in the assessment of the underpinning knowledge of anatomy and physiology tied into each competence (e.g. Jeffrey, 2000) and some units have ensured that these packages are successfully completed prior to the secondment on to a critical care course. Despite this, many teaching staff reported the need to revisit anatomy and physiology to redress any shortfall upon which subsequent teaching might be built (Scholes and Endacott, 2002). However, the competing demands for subject coverage within a limited taught programme have resulted in this material frequently being delivered through distance or self-directed learning packages which may not be directly assessed (ibid.). The notion that this area of applied knowledge will be rigorously assessed in practice by supervisors can be a faulty assumption, especially when the student is empowered to self-select an assessor and/or defend themselves from challenge.

combined with poor assessment of knowledge and skills in practice have all contributed to the failure to recognise and act upon earlier signs that the patient is becoming dangerously unwell (Chellel *et al.*, 2002).

During the allocation to critical care placements on the new curriculum, the students' poor grasp of anatomy and physiology and of pharmacology became very apparent. In many sites (Trusts and HEIs) remedial packages were prepared to redress the shortfall. This included onsite teaching sessions, learning packages and mini assessments. The allocation to the critical care environment brought home the amount of time the students needed to invest in studying this aspect of the curriculum to be safe in the setting. Many responded to this, but others found that competing demands, such as dead-lines for theoretical assessments, or completing their practice assessment documentation, could overwhelm their best intentions. Therefore, unless the mentor specifically pursued this aspect of the students' learning as part of their practice assessment (and in some cases the way that the competencies or learning outcomes were written made this difficult), students could progress through the placement without having redressed the shortfall in their know-ledge. Where students were on learning circuits, or worked with different mentors throughout their allocation, they were better able to defend them-selves from direct questioning and scrutiny by someone who had a sense of the progression and developments the student was making throughout the allocation. This led the team to conclude that: 'The amount of time dedicated to the delivery of applied physiology and pharmacology and the way this was tested in practice remains one of the weakest aspects in the new curriculum' (Executive Summary, Scholes *et al.*, 2004).

To enable the students to more effectively meet the needs of the critically sick patient in the acute care area, recommendations were made, namely that:

- A minimum time be specified to address physiology and anatomy within the curriculum.
- Formal assessment of applied physiology and the implications for clinical decision making be a requirement in all curricula.
- Simulated practice-based assessments such as Objective Structured Clin-ical Examinations (OSCEs)[5] be included to supplement other approaches to practice assessment.
- Qualified nurses be given prompts to help them focus the questioning of students to draw out their knowledge of applied physiology and the implications for patient assessment.

---

[5] OSCEs are a practical examination of students' competence in specific aspects of practice or task. They are run in circuits, each composed of a number of stations set up to test a candidate's response to a given simulation or scenario. In some cases this involves contact with a patient, actor, skills model or computer simulator. The assessor looks for precision as well as the underpinning knowledge to inform the assessee's performance. OSCEs are an exacting form of assessment, but are criticised because they only capture competence at the moment of assessment.

■ Consideration be given to the introduction of a fifth branch of nursing so that nurses wishing to practise either in acute and critical care environments or in primary care settings have adequate time to focus on curricular topics and spend time in placements that are most likely to develop the knowledge and skills that will impact upon their sphere of practice (Scholes *et al.*, 2004).

This contextual background raises some important issues for mentors/assessors to take into account when making a baseline assessment of the student's capabilities. In addition these issues will help the mentor/assessor consider how they might facilitate the student's transitional development whilst allocated to critical care.

Facilitating the student through the preparation and encounter phase of their allocation to critical care

First, there should be a thorough assessment of the student's expectations of the learning they might achieve whilst in the critical care environment including a review of:

■ The students' previous exposure to a critical care environment and/or past clinical experience caring for the acutely sick or rapidly deteriorating patient.
■ The match between the formal learning outcomes and/or clinical competencies set out in practice assessment documentation with the aspirational or personal learning goals of the student (seeking to illuminate areas of potential contradiction or confirmation). It is important for the mentor to help the student to focus upon the transferable skills that can be applied back to the recognition, assessment and care of the acutely ill patient in a general ward as well as the skills or competencies that they will need whilst allocated to critical care. In less traditional or novel 'critical care/ high dependency environments', where the acquisition of critical care skills may seem less obvious, it is essential that the mentor enable the students to identify learning from this experience that can inform the recognition, assessment and care of the acutely ill patient in a general ward.
■ The student's past experience and expectations of high support and high challenge. Establish from the outset that the student will be exposed to regular questioning and feedback and that they will be expected to question their mentor. Also establish with the student that they will be invited to identify the learning that has taken place each day as part of their shift debriefing.

Secondly, consideration must be given to the formal preparation the student has experienced for the allocation and how this has been integrated into their understanding of critical care nursing practice by:

■ Establishing the student's knowledge of baseline physiology to inform clinical decisions (a knowledge test might well be useful to help the student to identify the learning they need to instigate). A knowledge test is useful for the mentor because they are then fully aware of the baseline from which they are operating. Importantly, this would help to provide an agreed standard against which all students are judged and would help to improve parity and equivalence in assessment across the student cohort. Critically, sharing this knowledge assessment with the local college is important to reduce inequity in the assessment process but also to cross-check that there is not an unrealistic expectation of the student's knowledge and competence relative to their stage of development. The importance of this issue cannot be overstated, and it is an area of frequent tension that can arise between students, mentors and personal tutors.

■ Making explicit the learning opportunities from visits to specialist environments from the base unit. It may well be useful to guide the student and encourage them to focus on specific learning opportunities. After such visits it is important to help the student make sense of that learning and see how that can be applied back to acute and critical nursing situations. A useful tool is to ask the student to identify two elements of learning from their visit as a starting point to trigger purposive and critical reflection on the experience (this is not as easy as it sounds). After this the student should be encouraged to identify two action points for each one of those elements of learning (this may be further reading, exposure to new skills, or even new visits). But it is important to ensure that the student does apply their new knowledge or has the opportunity to rehearse or consolidate a clinical skill and does not simply become a tourist visiting new sites without making any sense of how these experiences inform their practice. Importantly, to ensure these action points have been pursued and that new learning has occurred, the mentor needs to probe and in some instances offer higher order questioning (see Fig. 7.2, p. 147).

Thirdly, locate the student into a social network or team within the unit. This can be achieved by:

■ Explicitly identifying the role expectation of students within the critical care environment, making known basic ground rules and parameters of performance and giving permission to the student to question and make known any concerns.

■ Helping the student to identify formal and informal networks of support within the unit and the different environmental (and emotional) zones within the unit.

■ Creating an open trusting rapport with the student that fosters the possibility of critical reflection but also the expression of feelings.

Finally, establish the centrality of the allocation to critical care to the student's projected career trajectory by asking the following:

- Is this an elective placement?
- Does the student intend to work in critical care once qualified?
- How does the student view the critical care environment in terms of informing their professional transition to qualified practitioner?
- How does the student view this allocation as part of their socialisation into a career as a lifelong learner?

The review thus far has illuminated critical issues that need to be addressed by the student and their mentor when the student is in the preparation or encounter phase of their transition. Many of the issues identified might be 'taken for granted'. Recent evidence suggests, however, that much of this initial diagnostic or baseline assessment is far from routine, and therefore it has been included here as a timely reminder. The next section explores factors that influence the adjustment phase in the transitional process: the power of socialisation and its impact on the learning process. This is explored, drawing on data from a study of student socialisation into A&E. Although the focus is specific to one environment, it illuminates key areas for consideration when working alongside students in any critical care environment, i.e. that before the student could **learn about** critical care nursing, they first had to **learn how to be** a critical care nursing student.

Socialisation and learning

A study of student nurses in the accident and emergency department was initiated by students' dichotomous evaluations of A&E as an environment they either 'loved' or 'hated' (Scholes, 1988). One cohort of students was followed, capturing their initial expectations of the A&E allocation whilst in school, and was followed through with periods of observation of their experience in A&E and subsequently their evaluations of the experience in the reflective block after the allocation.[6]

Expectations of the experience

Personal experience of A&E, or accounts from family members or friends, were found to be very powerful in shaping the students' expectations of their experience. But of greater influence was media representation of A&E. This can

---

[6] The student cohort was made up of 24 students who were programmed to be allocated to A&E in the third year of their training. Of these students 15 were observed in practice working alongside their mentors. Informal interviews were conducted with the students whilst in the field. Analysis of the students' curriculum, timetable and practice assessment documentation was undertaken in order to examine the learning outcomes which were set out to guide the students' learning in the A&E department. The conclusion was that socialisation was the gateway to learning (Scholes, 1988).

include soap operas, dramas or documentary films, all edited for maximum audience effect and therefore portraying a somewhat dramatic account of real life in an A&E department. Nevertheless their power to affect students' expectations of the experience and to raise anxiety about the allocation should not be underestimated (Kalisch and Kalisch, 1986).

Fundamentally, students were of the impression that A&E predominantly dealt with very sick patients; interventions needed to be speedy; any disease, mental illness or trauma could bring a patient to the department; and patients cut across the whole lifespan. As such, students felt that they would need a very wide range of knowledge and skills to meet the needs of patients attending A&E. In addition, students were anxious about having to interact with a whole range of health care professionals such as community psychiatric nurses (CPNs), medical specialists, dentists and paramedics, social workers, the police, voluntary workers, and other staff whom they may not have encountered before.

At the time of the study, the students wore hats with stripes depicting the number of years they had completed in training. Students were allocated to A&E at the beginning of their third year. They were concerned about what would be expected of them because of their third-year stripe, i.e. they felt that they would be assumed to have a reasonable grasp of knowledge and range of skills but that they were being allocated to an area of practice that was quite different from anything they had encountered before. With all these considerations in mind, students had considerable anxiety about starting their placement. These considerations have been summarised in Table 5.1 to demonstrate the range of factors that impacted upon their expectations of the experience using the transitional model (Allen and van de Vliert, 1984).

Initial behaviours on the A&E placement

When the students arrived on their first day, many felt paralysed by their anxiety and the intrinsic uncertainty or potential threats inherent within the department. They were clear about one thing: anything could happen. Therefore, they had to learn to position themselves within the team and within the geography of the unit to avoid unnecessary exposure to difficult situations. This had been clearly outlined in school and was reinforced by their mentors.

Students therefore had to invest time in working out how they should behave in the department. This could be divided into three phases: the first, shortest and most painful stage for the student was when they had to 'fumble about' in the department acclimatising themselves to the environment. In some cases this also served to keep the student away from the patients and the staff as they invested considerable energy and effort into examining cupboards, the sluice or office. During this period they 'stumbled upon' pieces of information or a qualified member of staff who would then direct them specifically to what they should do next. Once they had grasped the basic principles of what they should do, they could then work more actively to

Table 5.1 Student nurses' expectations of A&E prior to their placement.

Antecedent conditions	Factors that impacted upon expectations
Chance events	Experience of A&E as a patient or relative
	Images created by media – risk of exposure to: ■ traumatic events, complicated by drugs and alcohol ■ horrific injuries, sudden death ■ infested clients, profoundly disturbed or aggressive clients, self-harmers ■ violence directed towards the staff ■ high levels of distress among relatives
Societal forces	Waiting time targets – trolley waits Triage management Media depiction of quality of care in A&E Uncontrolled volume of patients dependent on incidents – minimal locus of control
Changes in roles senders	Media depiction – reality of experience Range of different professionals with whom they needed to interact Image of the A&E nurse Speed of interactions
Change in capabilities or motives of the role sender	Practice development initiatives Mentoring/practice educators/lecturer practitioners/role models Learning outcomes/competencies for placement Academic assignments to be completed whilst on placement
Change in capabilities or motives of the focal person	Third-year-stripe syndrome Past experience with critically ill patients Knowledge development – potential to learn a range of new skills and knowledge Personal preferences, ambitions for career Life experiences in coping with alternative lifestyles

seek direction. Some did this in a canny way, by situating themselves next to the white board, a position from which they knew they would be directed, whilst others were more proactive and actively sought out key people who would offer guidance.

For the first time since they started their training, students had to situate themselves so they could be directed by the shift leader to do a specific activity and report back. Until such time as this was clearly understood and demonstrated, the student would be called back to the central point of organisation.[7] For many students, it was unusual to have to report back the minutiae of their interactions and findings to the person in charge. The students needed to understand that it was critical for the shift leader to know where the students were, what they were doing and that they could be relied upon to bring back relevant information about the patient: that they were the eyes and ears of the shift leader and this was how the shift leader could keep the department running smoothly.

'Fitting in'

Students were not only assessed on *whether* they did this, but on *how they did it* as well. The qualified staff in the A&E department moved with deliberation and speed to keep pace with the busy workload. Also staff had to be focused and purposive and to distil the relevant information from patients and pass this on to the shift leader. Some students found it hard to be so assiduous, especially when they were inhibited by their anxiety. Others did manage to do this, and when this was the case they were said to 'manifest the right attitude'. If they did this, they were 'fostered' by the A&E staff and taken into situations of increasing diversity and allowed to use their own initiative (on the proviso that they still reported back what they were doing and where they were in the department). Exposure to a range of patients with different needs matched the students' expectations about what could be learnt from A&E. In addition, the freedom to demonstrate this initiative fitted with their expectations of their third-year status. They found the experience exciting and expanding and they 'loved it'.

Conversely, students who did not demonstrate the 'right attitude', by being too hard, too cynical, too soft or too slow, or who seemed generally uninterested or suspected of disingenuous motives, never progressed from the point of returning to the A&E board and being told to go and 'ob and undress' the next patient. For them, the experience was evaluated as either 'tedious and boring' or 'nerve wracking and unpleasant'.

The transparency of either 'fitting in' and thereby being accepted as a member of the subcultural world, or failing to do so and thereby being excluded was extremely obvious. However, the staff were clear that a tight ship was essential to keep the department working effectively. Furthermore, patient and staff safety could be at risk unless there was compliance, and therefore there was very little tolerance within the system for self-expression. The conclusion was drawn that **to learn about** A&E nursing one first had **to learn how to be** a student nurse in A&E (Scholes, 1988).

---

[7] The white board listed the patients in the department and a brief outline of key investigations, diagnosis or expected patient destination. It was a central position to which all staff returned to report back information or to pick up new work. This is powerfully conveyed in the television drama 'ER', but these data preceded that series.

Although these data are now quite historic, and despite two major reviews of the pre-registration curriculum, countless reports, and policy recommendations to enhance the quality of practice learning, the findings from this study hold a contemporary message. Students may now see 'fitting in' and demonstrating 'the right attitude' as a thing of the past but do so at their peril. A number of studies have shown that 'demonstrating the right attitude' crucially influenced the assessment of the student (e.g. Melia, 1981; Girot, 1993; Phillips *et al.*, 2000: 72). However, some Project 2000 students embraced the idea that they were students of the university rather than students of the Trust[8], an issue that the Peach Report recommendations sought to redress (UKCC, 1999). Within partnership working, Trust representatives powerfully argued that student punctuality and attendance, professional presentation of self and engagement in practice were areas that required significant attention. Many encouraged the HEIs to produce assessment documents that specifically identified these areas, and, if a student was continually late, dishevelled and requesting periods of absence from the clinical area, this was a point of practice failure. It was thus made clear that demonstrating 'the right attitude' was about respect for colleagues and patients and about conveying an identity of professionalism (Scholes *et al.*, 2004). This issue is examined in greater detail in Chapter 7.

It is therefore important at the outset of any allocation for the mentor to make explicit the 'ground rules' and stated behavioural norms for the student on that placement. Even when this is made explicit, the student has to establish (as part of the socialisation process in the adjustment phase of their transition):

- to whom they might safely direct a question (this might not be their mentor, especially if they are also an assessor);
- how to frame questions and when to ask them;
- whom they can trust to impart 'sound' knowledge and skills;
- how to pace their efforts.

Each environment will have a set of implicit social norms that frequently go unstated. Creating the opportunity in which a student can declare any deficit in competence or experience (by offering an amnesty on such declarations) is critical to ensure that no question is left unspoken, especially where this could affect patient safety. Most critical care environments do encourage students to ask questions and do 'nothing' unless a qualified nurse is present or they have been assessed as competent. Although such instruction seems straightforward,

---

[8] Being a student of the university and under the banner of supernumerary status was assumed by some students as giving them licence to absent themselves from practice if they did not consider suitable learning opportunities were on offer in favour of following up their studies 'in the library'. Furthermore, complaints from practitioners, patients and their relatives about some students' choice of self-expression through dress, jewellery and hairstyles were on the increase. Many practitioners and educationalists were concerned about the negative image this gave of the profession and were enthusiastic to see this behaviour acknowledged as unacceptable.

the student has to 'test' the veracity of this throughout the adjustment phase of their transition. For example, how literal is 'doing nothing'? What questions can be asked of whom without invoking criticism? Where should the student stand; what of their posture and gait? How do they appear interested when they are unable to engage in clinical care? A negative response can extinguish the student's questioning or inhibit their willingness to engage fully with their qualified mentors. It most certainly will limit their willingness to take intellectual risks and place themselves in learning situations which might expose weakness in their knowledge or ability. However, although all these factors may seem to build a case for not having students in critical care environments, it should be remembered that:

- The students are learning the skills to recognise, assess and act to meet the needs of the deteriorating patient, hence the investment in such learning will affect patient outcome and timely admission and discharge from critical care environments.
- Exposure to positive and encouraging mentors is a key variable in the recruitment and retention of critical care staff.
- Investment in the student experience pays dividends as the input at this stage will be rewarded by colleagues in the future with the appropriate knowledge and skills to make an effective contribution to the team.

The exploration thus far has been on how to enable pre-registration students. The text now turns to review how to support and facilitate colleagues undertaking post-registration education in critical care.

Post-registration education in critical care

The chapter now addresses socialising forces within academic settings and the impact these have had on formal learning programmes about critical care nursing. This is done through the theoretical lens of 'McDonaldization' (Ritzer, 1996).[9] The impact of this on the provision of post-registration critical care education in the UK is analysed.[10] The conclusion is drawn that stakeholder demands for greater efficiency in post-registration education provision

---

[9] Although the arguments on which these issues were raised came through a research study into post-registration provision of critical care education, the issues are significant for pre-registration preparation as well.

[10] This analysis is based on an evaluation of the effectiveness of the former ENB critical care courses for intensive care, coronary care, theatre and anaesthetic, A&E, and paediatric intensive care nursing. Subsequently these programmes have been amalgamated into the critical care portfolio or pathways provided by HEI providers. However, the study of the former ENB clinical courses illuminated some critical issues that impact on critical care students' experiences within HEIs, and the tensions that the new mode of educational provision might have upon the learning experiences of students.

can fundamentally contradict notions of effective learning. Therefore, these contextual factors will ultimately impact upon student attitude and commitment to their learning encounters, and need to be considered when attempting to facilitate the transition of colleagues towards expertise.

Socialisation in education: the case in post-registration programmes[11]

'McDonaldization' is a term used by Ritzer (1996) to present a modern-day image of Weber's classic construct of rationalisation and the bureaucratic structure. Ritzer argues that McDonalds' economic organisation, with efficiency and effectiveness at its heart, has been widely adopted across a range of services and in the production of goods (Smart, 1999). Further, he argues that principles of economic organisation (efficiency, continuity of operations, speed, precision and calculation of results – the driving goals of rationality) have now influenced higher education and health. This influence can be detected in all but the most resistant cultures around the world (Ritzer, 1996). The impact of market principles on non-profit-making organisations can be explained using the McDonaldization thesis (Smart, 1999). In this context it will be used to examine the outcome of such change for the provision of post-registration critical care education in the UK and the implications for the future preparation of critical care practitioners.

The Higher Education Sector has had to respond to wider societal demands for efficiency, predictability, calculability and control. In part this has been essential to adapt to the 'massification' (Trow, 1973) of the sector. Indeed, the Government's target to have 50% of the population under the age of 30 engaged in some way in higher education by 2010 (DfEE, 1998) indicates greater challenges ahead.

Since the introduction of the quasi purchaser/provider split (Francis and Humphrey, 1998), courses are now viewed as purchased products. As such, they are frequently discussed using terminology normally associated with retail or business, e.g. convenience, efficiency, effectiveness, and value for money. Content is determined on the basis of what makes the course attractive to the purchaser. By reducing education into accessible chunks the criterion of convenience is met. Providing access to a wide range of available goods (modules) of uniform quality (credit rating) fulfils the efficiency criterion, especially when they are intensively delivered through economy of scale. However, a system set in place to find the solution to one set of problems raises a new set of challenges.

---

[11] **Acknowledgement**. This section of the chapter is based on research undertaken by the author and her colleague, Professor Ruth Endacott. The evaluation was funded by the English National Board of Nursing, Midwifery and Health Visiting. All views expressed in this section, except those reported as data, are those of the researchers.

Table 5.2 Comparison between the 'fast food' principles and current course delivery.

Fast food principles	Course delivery
Variety in the basic product provided by 'add on' items/flavours	A menu of module options within a programme 'pathway'
Quick and convenient way to satiate hunger	Learning material selected and provided for the student based on service need or specified competencies
Good value for money	Students released for taught time only or self-funded
Cheap product achieved through economy of scale	Courses only run when student numbers are viable/economical – larger cohorts favoured
Taste and quality predictable wherever it is purchased in the world	Comparable outcomes and credits for specific courses and academic awards, calls for greater parity and equivalence in student abilities

Modularised courses are delivered using standardised contact hours for credit rating and this can result in less attention being devoted to whether a given subject is best taught in that time (Ritzer, 2000: 66). Over three decades ago Parlett (1969) cautioned that time restrictions in programme delivery make a learner more syllabus bound. However, this might be considered a positive outcome through a 'McDonaldization' lens because it ensures greater standardisation. Furthermore, this approach fits with a perception that: 'a lot of something, or the quick delivery of it means it must be good' (Ritzer, 2000: 12). However, when this is analysed in greater depth, it can be seen that such an assumption is wrong (Smart, 1999). Table 5.2 makes comparisons between the retail principles of fast food and current course delivery.

In the context of education: how do efficiency and effectiveness, flexibility and choice actually affect the quality of the learning experience and academic integrity? Brookfield (1984) contested that as more adult learners come into the system with varying learning styles and personalities, and with different past professional experiences and abilities, it is crucial to individualise the curriculum to maximise learning potential. However, current systems militate against individualisation. As such, education can become a dehumanising experience, especially when there are large cohorts of students with minimal time for personal tutorials and reduced opportunities to share with each other (Ritzer, 2000: 143). Grouping students together and lecturing at them, especially when the lecturer is not inspirational, may be cost and resource efficient, but is learning inefficient (Brook, 1994). Sessions can become clock-watching exercises which may *occupy* the student without *engaging them* in the process (Ritzer, 2000) or without stimulating them to apply new learning back to the clinical setting.

For nearly a decade, HEIs have had to balance the tension of providing courses which offer maximum flexibility, choice and convenience at the lowest possible cost yet which yield the most profitable outcomes (Scholes and Endacott, 2002). But the perspective on what constituted a profitable outcome varied according to the 'professional lens' through which you viewed the issue. For example, the student might evaluate on the basis of certification, managers on the basis of risk reduction and quality assurance, and workforce planners using criteria of speed and value for money. When analysing various stakeholders' perceptions of what made a critical care course effective, one can see a diverse set of issues.

Students defined the course as effective if:

- it enhanced their understanding of patients' conditions and or relevant clinical activities;
- they learnt something new that enhanced their understanding of the speciality (e.g. the wider policy context);
- it enabled them to participate in the multiprofessional health care team with greater confidence.

Educationalists held different views. 'Effectiveness' of a course meant that students underwent:

- a significant transition or awakening to their therapeutic potential as critical care practitioners; or
- an educational experience that would enable them to challenge the status quo, critically review their own practice and take measures to develop practice in the setting and/or assist in the development of others.

In terms of maximising the effectiveness of a course, some considered that a supernumerary period that allowed the student to practise in units other than their work base was essential.[12] Others considered that continued experience in their original work base was more effective on the proviso that they worked alongside a skilled supervisor who used the practice assessment tool to its full potential. However, many educationalists held grave doubts that mentors were assessing students with consistent rigour and robustness; and subsequent research has demonstrated that this is not a problem unique to the critical care setting (e.g. Duffy, 2003; Scholes *et al.*, 2004). How to effect learning and transitions through assessment is examined in Chapter 7.

Managers' views also varied. They suggested that a course was effective when it: enabled the acquisition of new skills whilst on the course or allowed for the consolidation of existing skills and the examination of research evidence

---

[12] It is of interest, that as this has become less likely, staff development programmes have taken up rotation programmes to expand staff's repertoire of skills. Please see Chapter 6.

to support those activities. In many instances the number of staff who held the ENB award was presented as a quality marker for the unit, and the offer of a place on the course was used in their recruitment and retention strategy. Some managers felt that time invested in study leave for a student to undertake a clinical experience on another unit was worthwhile, and this was rewarded if and when the student was able to bring back fresh ideas to their base unit. Most, however, considered a course **efficient** if it minimally disrupted service provision or staffing levels (i.e. did not disrupt productivity). This latter position is now the dominant voice. In response, work-based learning and on-line and distance-learning programmes have been devised.

Finally, many stakeholders believed a course was only effective when it was responsive to local need and rapid change. As a consequence they were more resistant to the introduction of national threshold standards or core competencies for the critical care programmes because they feared this might inhibit local flexibility. Therefore, when attempting to gain agreement of what constituted core competencies as an outcome of the former ENB critical care courses, the diversity and complexity of provision made agreement on the necessity for specific competencies problematic (Scholes and Endacott, 2002). An analysis of curriculum documentation of the critical care courses (formerly identified as ENB clinical courses) demonstrated that there was indeed wide interpretation of the outcomes for these programmes (Scholes *et al.*, 1999). Agreement could be reached if the competency was written as an abstract statement, but this resulted in wider individual interpretation which compromised standardisation and consistency (Scholes and Endacott, 2002). The factors leading to this diversity are now critically examined in light of current trends in academic provision.

Fundamental changes have affected post-registration clinical education. Students with varying levels of experience form heterogeneous groups. They remain in their work base for the practice element of the programme and undertake 'part-time' studies in college. This affects learning in three ways:

(1)   time for study;
(2)   student status; and
(3)   the prioritisation of learning product over learning process.

Time for study

The research data highlighted that the amount of time made available to the students to do their courses was variable (Scholes and Endacott, 2002). Recruitment and retention problems were often cited as the main cause of this. Some students were only given 50% of taught time in university as study leave whilst others were all but supernumerary throughout the whole programme.[13] The reduction in available study leave meant that more students could be put through courses, even though it was recognised that this could have less

---

[13] These data were collected in the period between spring 2000 and summer 2002.

effective outcomes for student learning. Alternatively, the time to complete the programme was reduced as a means of maintaining a high throughput. Here the dominant agenda was volume and spread of involvement rather than effective provision because recruitment and retention had priority.

However, in one site, theatre managers had found that this strategy had been so detrimental in effecting professional development that they reduced the number seconded to the course from all the partner Trusts and located all the students in one unit to intensify support. Alumnae were then on contract to work for their Trust for one year or incur a financial penalty. This system seemed to have a positive impact on retention, but the managers acknowledged that this was a local solution to resolve high staff turnover. These examples illustrate the way in which education has become a commodity with learning viewed more as a product (the qualification, the retention of staff) rather than a process (learning, the development of the individual student).

Post-registration 'student' status

The conferment of student status in practice fundamentally affected opportunities for learning within the clinical setting. For some, being a student only referred to time spent in college, whereas in practice their role did not change. Therefore, the amount of time the 'student' had to apply their theory to new situations and respond to the familiar being rendered strange by exposure to novel clinical situations could be seriously compromised because they were fully engaged in service delivery. Furthermore, collegiate relationships affected the assessment of practice. How could one assess or challenge a colleague who was deemed competent one day, when the next they were a 'course student' presenting a practice assessment document? This was termed the **practitioner–student gap** (Endacott *et al.*, 2003). To cope with the potential dissonance of this situation, students had to construct their learner status as only applicable to the academic setting: they inhabited two quite distinct communities, one academic and one in practice that had different foci, values and conceptions of learning and being a learner (Lave and Wenger, 1991; Wenger, 1998).

Learning product over learning process

Some clinicians suggested that part of the criteria for sending staff to do the course was based upon their competent performance in post. Furthermore, a solution for overstretched staff was to bypass practice assessment on the assumption that the individual was already competent before they did the programme. For these stakeholders the programme was more about the acquisition of academic outcomes rather than clinical competencies, and academic outcomes need not be assessed in practice.

This suggests that what you can do in the job (clinical competence) is given greater value than what you can learn from a course (practice learning outcomes/practice competencies). It also contrasts with the course intentions when these clinical programmes were at their peak, first as Joint Board for Clinical Nursing Studies (JBCNS) courses and, before their demise, as ENB numbered programmes. These programmes were primarily undertaken *before* the practitioner entered the speciality and were there to prepare the nurses for their role in clinical practice (Kite, 1998). They required a nurse to either be seconded or resign and take up her student role in a hospital where the programme was run. However, the courses could not keep up with demand, and wider access into programmes was achieved by enabling practitioners to stay in their workplace and attend HEIs for the theoretical component of the course. This meant that nurses were entering critical care environments without any formal preparation for the speciality, hence the introduction of D grade competency packages to redress this gap. The critical care course then became something other and in some instances lost its grip on what type of preparation clinicians felt was appropriate (Crunden, 1998). This moved the critical care community to demand greater standardisation of the clinical programmes, and to sharpen the focus of course content on matters of clinical competency. However, practitioners who had been through the courses understood that they were developmental and enhanced the professional performance of the nurse, but this was less easily definable than assessment against competences and standards of what could be done in the job. Harnessing this ambiguity, and then promising to deliver employees who were fit for purpose and practice through the use of clearly definable competences, the workforce planners have restructured critical care preparation.[14] Their strategies are promulgated as more cost effective with the advantage of minimising disruption to service provision. Under the umbrella of efficiency and effectiveness, and greater assurance of the standardisation of the product (quality assurance of the critical care practitioner), competencies have taken centre stage. Furthermore, they have been used to implement the modernisation agenda and to redefine the workforce (see Chapter 9). Some of the issues this raises are set out in Table 5.3.

Standardising educational competencies for critical care

The ambition to standardise competencies and quality assure a minimum standard of practice is a chimera, unless the minimum standard is set to accommodate the lowest common denominator which then means the goal is not ambitious. Why should this be the case? The first reason is that there is variability in the work base in which a practitioner can practise; and secondly, achieving consensus as to what constitutes **core competencies** remains contested.

---

[14] Looking through the McDonaldization lens this describes a requirement for education to be delivered at maximum speed with minimal disruption to the service and yet retain the quality of the product. Our study revealed some damaging outcomes from such an approach. Students who felt disenchanted by their experiences would feed back negative accounts of their course to the managers and commissioners, who then called for greater efficiency and more effective courses (Scholes and Endacott, 2002). However, systems set in place to furnish the need for efficiency, convenience, accessibility and standardisation seemed to be in contradiction to notions of what enabled effective learning.

Table 5.3 Comparison between the 'fast food' principles and competencies.

Fast food principles	Competencies
Variety in the basic product provided by 'add on' items/flavours	Additional competencies allocated to practitioners who provide a broader range of services. New services can be designed where no one meets the competencies with staff trained and assessed to meet the need
Quick and convenient way to satiate hunger	Immediate recognition of competencies and identification of the need for further developments. Greater control in determining what is needed for the job and what the individual can do to meet that. Competencies can be independent of professional background, therefore not dependent on prolonged professional education programmes to resource service delivery
Good value for money	Assessment takes place in the workplace, therefore you get what you want. Staff are paid for what they can do. Up-skilling of staff means that less expensive personnel can provide a service if deemed competent to fulfil the task
Cheap product achieved through economy of scale	In this case 'cost savings' made by providing in-house or work-based learning and not having to back-fill staff on courses
Taste and quality predictable wherever product is purchased in the world	National competencies assure a minimum standard

Variation in the experiences that a practitioner can acquire has arisen because patient dependency differed considerably from one unit to the next. The Audit Commission (1999) and the Department of Health (DH, 2000) determined that intensive care environments should be providing levels of care appropriate to patients with the greatest levels of dependency, and these needed to be distinguished from high dependency units where care was provided for patients with less complex and dependent needs. However, at the time of the ENB research, students were coming from units with highly variable provision (Scholes and Endacott, 2002). Therefore, trying to agree on core competencies as outcomes from the clinical courses was problematic. An example was a competency linked to caring for a patient on haemofiltration. Some units rarely used haemofiltration and therefore did not consider this 'core'. In units where haemofiltration was commonplace, it was considered essential. Hence some students might not be able to achieve certain competencies if they stayed in their work base. This was termed the **practice–competency**

gap (Scholes and Endacott, 2003). The easiest solution was to drop the notion of the competency as 'core', but this did not satisfy those who were seeking the use of core competencies to raise the minimum national standard.

Work-based assessment of competence might redress this issue, but fundamentally does not resolve the problem of local variation in provision. This variation in practice experience could be logged in a portfolio, and increasingly the portfolio could have a more significant role in supporting claims of competence made by applicants to new posts. However, the capacity of written media to convey what an individual can do is notoriously unreliable (Endacott *et al.*, 2003). Furthermore, although it is important to know that the individual is not competent to manage haemofiltration, it does not resolve the problem for employers who want them to be able to do this. Managers might be reluctant to invest their own resources in up-skilling that individual to meet a competence they consider core, pushing the cost back on to the individual practitioner. Such a practice would require careful and robust professional regulation to ensure practitioners and patients were not disadvantaged or placed at risk by hard-nosed employers taking short cuts to savings.

Implications for future provision of critical care education

The agenda for future provision is being shaped by ideals of increased efficiency, greater predictability (calls for greater standardisation and replication from one setting to the next), greater calculability (cost, time it takes to get the product, risk management) and control (who gets what and for what purpose). Such values were espoused because of a genuine concern to minimally disrupt the service and to achieve maximum access to an educational experience. However, greater standardisation has a predisposition to settle for the lowest common denominator of provision, rather than leading to an aspirational attempt to raise the bar of expectation. Using the language of the market, if what was on sale was not to the purchaser's requirements or taste, the response was to turn to in-house provision and assessment of what the individual could do in the job expressed as outcome-standard-based statements, or competencies. This has the potential to drive a wedge between the academic provider and the service. In response, HEI providers have had to reposition themselves and restructure their provision, at times in great haste. This repositioning has been politically driven by 'popularity'-based policy (Watson and Bowden, 2005) which is further complicated by the competing demands from the sector's different stakeholders. At times this has led to chaotic outfall, especially for the students on courses, which can potentially create further alienation from the HEI sector and a stronger desire to provide 'in-house' or work-based solutions.

The critical issue is that what seems to be a quick and easy solution (in-house study days, more work-based learning) may in the longer term be as faulty as that which preceded it, if the causes of the original problem are not addressed (considering learning theories, learning styles, and ways to achieve effective practice-based learning). Such an issue needs careful consideration (by academics and clinicians) when introducing the continuing professional development agenda of the 'skills escalator' (DH, 2002). (Approaches to maximise the potential of such learning experiences are examined in Chapter 6.) If we continue to pay scant regard to how people learn and just assume that they will by exposure to the latest educational medium, we face a pretty dismal future.[15] What is more depressing is that so many educationalists, clinicians and students are becoming frustrated and disenfranchised from the business of teaching, simply because the demands of the system require them to work in a way that inhibits them from applying the core principles of learning theory. Just as we are now seeing a movement towards the restoration of core professional values and standards in clinical practice, one hopes to see a similar movement rise up among nurse academics who reposition themselves as educators for clinical practice, not solely educators whose purpose is to process the requisite number of students and enable them to achieve a set of minimal academic outcomes.

In the current provision of post-registration critical care education the purchaser is not the primary consumer of the course. Workforce planners may see little value in sending students on a course, and press for further reductions in time and speed in getting results. But they are not the individual going through that process. There are greater freedoms and potential for creativity for those high in the bureaucracy (commissioning education) but there is a need for them to exert greater control and require greater predictability over those they manage (Ritzer, 2000: 118). Therefore, the needs of those who do (course members) may well be at odds with the values of those who commission, although so pervasive are the phenomena of the McDonaldization process that the student can echo the immediate benefits of the system without sight of the longer term disadvantages. The pragmatic stance of immediacy and convenience may attract future students and their managers, rather than the promise of a programme which might have longer term implications for transformed knowledge and practice. Although nursing has some unique dilemmas, some of those contradictions are shared by others providing vocational and professional education (Zukas and Malcolm, 2002).

Since the Scholes and Endacott (2002) study a number of initiatives have been implemented that have had a significant impact on provision. The ENB clinical courses no longer exist, and, as has already been illustrated, have been absorbed by the HEI portfolio of critical care programmes within pathways leading to an academic award. Secondly, while the widespread appointment

---

[15] New modes of delivery to enhance flexibility including distance, on-line and work-based learning (as opposed to in-house or in-service competency development) are strongly advocated (Audit Commission, 1999). Although these modes of delivery have been reviewed as effective means to enhance professional development, as yet we do not have any robust research to indicate how these approaches transform clinical practice.

of practice educators and critical care nurse consultants was only just emerging at the time of the research, it has now done much to redress concerns about practice learning and stimulated a far more concerted effort in fostering professional development. The focus on enhancing the quality and rigour of practice assessment, clinical supervision and mentoring has become a central agenda for the NMC (ENB/DH, 2001a,b; Asbridge, 2003). However, the fragmentation of formal educational experiences for post-registration critical care students remains an issue. Although there is a drive for Strategic Health Authorities to commission education that serves to realise practice-based outcomes, and a move to map Agenda for Change competencies in with formal educational provision (McLean *et al.*, 2005), the longer term impact of these in achieving transformed practice knowledge requires robust evaluation.

Factors to consider when facilitating learning transitions in colleagues

In light of this contextual backdrop, the following issues need to be considered when supporting colleagues undertaking post-registration education programmes.

First, a thorough assessment of the student's expectations and exploration of how they intend to apply their new learning from a course back into their professional practice. This will include:

- A review of the learning outcomes or competencies and translation into learning opportunities within clinical practice or consolidation of skills for the clinical context.
- A review of the student's expectations of high support and high challenge, especially if their assessor or mentor is a colleague. Review who should undertake this role, to ensure their relative positional authority and knowledge of that mentor/assessor, but also consider on-site deliberative exploration of the issues as they are applied in a nursing context, i.e. what is to be assessed by whom and under what circumstances. Notice any learner who defends themselves from any learning which might trigger contradiction or who constantly locates themselves in safe situations (i.e. avoiding continuity in their chosen assessor or seeking fragmented experiences or multiple visits without exploring the meaning of this learning to their practice).

Secondly, a review of the student's knowledge to inform clinical decisions should be undertaken. The mentor/assessor should take into consideration the impact of new learning on contradicting past assumptions which can invoke serious questions about fundamental skills and competence. This may cause a significant loss in confidence for the post-registration student, whilst they assimilate their new knowledge into their repertoire of performance. This can be assessed by the following means.

- Check out areas of contradiction by explicitly asking the students to articulate areas of new learning from a programme. Reinforce the notion of their 'student status' whilst on the course to allow them to take intellectual risks and invest in a wide range of learning opportunities.
- Offer amnesty to address fundamental competence and knowledge, and identify if new learning has exposed weakness in foundational understanding. Sharing one's own experience of this can enable a student to feel confident to disclose these areas.
- Ensure the student has adequate supervision in times of crises in confidence.

Thirdly, locate the students in a social network or team within the unit that is supportive of learners. The facilitator needs to consider whether:

- this might be best effected by allocating a post-registration student to a new clinical team, and one that is particularly supportive of learners;
- they have created an open trusting rapport with the student that fosters the possibility of critical reflection but also the expression of feelings.

Finally, establish the centrality of this new learning to their career trajectories and where they might focus rehearsal and consolidation of new learning.

As more and more education and training are taking place in the workplace for learners outside formal educational programmes, the next two chapters offer strategies and models of support to best effect learning transitions in colleagues.

References

Akinsanya J (1985) Learning about life. *Senior Nurse* **2**: 24–25.

Allen V and van de Vliert E (1984) *Role Transitions: Explorations and Explanations.* NATO Conference Series. Series III: Human Factors. New York: Plenum Press.

Asbridge J (2003) Speech to the RCN Annual Congress. Downloaded from: www.Rcn.org.news/congress 2003/display.php?ID=491&Highlight=1 (accessed 15 March 2005).

Audit Commission (1999) *Critical to Success. The Place of Efficient and Effective Critical Care Services within the Acute Hospital.* London: Audit Commission.

Barker M (1996) Should there be a nursing presence in the operating theatre? *British Journal of Nursing* **5**(18): 1134–1137.

Brook N (1994) A sharp intake of breath: inspirations in education – some of the issues. *Physiotherapy* **81**(9): 506–513.

Brookfield S (1984) *Adult Learners, Adult Education and the Community.* Open University Press, Milton Keynes.

Carberry M (2002) Implementing the modified early warning system: our experiences. *Nursing in Critical Care* **7**(5): 220–226.

Chellel A, Fraser J and Fender V (2002) Nursing observations on ward patients at risk of critical illness with outreach nurses in Kent. *Nursing Times* **98**(46): 36–39.

Coad S, Haines S and Lawrence B (2002) Supporting ward staff in acute areas: the past, present and the future? *Nursing in Critical Care* **7**(3): 126–131.

Conway J (1995) A monkey can do your job! *British Journal of Theatre Nursing* **5**(9): 12–15, 31.

Crunden E (1998) Developing a strategy to facilitate the effective preparation of nurses for specialist practice. Paper delivered at Providing Education for Practice, BACCN Annual Conference, Manchester, 20–22 October.

Department for Education and Employment (DfEE) (1998) *Higher Education in the 21st Century*. London: HMSO.

Department of Health (1999) *Making a Difference, Strengthening the Nursing, Midwifery and Health Visiting Contribution to Health and Healthcare*. London: DH.

Department of Health (2000) *Comprehensive Critical Care. A Review of Adult Critical Care Services*. London: DH.

Department of Health (2001) *The Nursing Contribution to the Provision of Comprehensive Critical Care for Adults. A Strategic Programme of Action*. PL CNO 2001 10: London: HMSO.

Department of Health (2002) The Skills Escalator. www.doh.gov.uk/hrinthenhs/learning/ (accessed 15 January 2005).

Department of Health and NHS Modernisation Agency (2003) *Critical Care Outreach 2003: Progress in Developing Services*. London: DH and NHS Modernisation Agency.

Duffy K (2003) *Failing Students: A Qualitative Study of Factors that Influence the Decisions Regarding the Assessment of Students' Competence to Practise*. Glasgow: Caledonian Nursing and Midwifery Research Centre, Glasgow Caledonian University.

Durston M and Rance A (1995) Bridging the theory–practice gap in the ITU with in-service education. *Intensive Care Nursing* **11**: 233–236.

Endacott R, Scholes J, Freeman M and Cooper S (2003) The reality of clinical learning in critical care settings: a practitioner–student gap? *Journal of Clinical Nursing* **12**: 778–785.

English National Board for Nursing, Midwifery and Health Visiting/Department of Health (2001a) *Placements in Focus*. ENB/DH: London.

English National Board for Nursing, Midwifery and Health Visiting/Department of Health (2001b) *Preparation for Mentors and Teachers. A New Framework of Guidance*. ENB/DH: London.

Eraut M, Alderton J, Boylan A and Wraight A (1995) *Learning to Use Scientific Knowledge in Education and Practice Settings: an Evaluation of the Contribution of the Biological, Behavioural and Social Sciences to Pre-registration Nursing and Midwifery Programmes*. London: ENB.

Francis B and Humphrey J (1998) Education or centralisation? Differences in the development of nurse education commissioning policy among UK nations. *Nurse Education Today* **18**(6): 433–439.

Garrard C and Young D (1998) Sub-optimal care of patients before admission to intensive care. *British Medical Journal* **318**: 53–54.

Girot E (1993) Assessment of competence in clinical practice: a phenomenological approach. *Journal of Advanced Nursing* **18**: 114–119.

Goldhill D, Worthington L, Mulcahy A, Tarling M and Summer A (1999) The patient at risk team: identifying and managing seriously ill patients. *Anaesthesia* **54**: 853–860.

Jeffrey Y (2000) Using competencies to promote a learning environment in intensive care. *Nursing in Critical Care* **5**(4): 194–198.

Institute of Employment Studies (2003) *1st Year Survey, The Evaluation of Nurse Education Partnerships; 3rd Year Survey for the Evaluation of Nurse Education Partnerships; Repeat 1st Year Survey for the Evaluation of Nurse Education Partnerships*. Sussex: Institute of Employment Studies.

Jones C (1990) The Bevan Report: Comments Sent by the Chairman to Mrs Ann Poole, Chief Nursing Officer at the DHSS on behalf of the NATN, in response to the recent publication of the Bevan Report. *British Journal of Theatre Nursing* **27**(3): 9.

Kalisch P and Kalisch B (1986) A comparative analysis of nurse and physician characters in the media. *Journal of Advanced Nursing* **11**: 176–195.

Kenward G and Hodgetts T (2002) Nurse concern: a predictor of patient deterioration. *Nursing Times* **98**(22): 38–39.

Kite K (1998) Learning to doubt: the professional development of nurses in one intensive therapy unit. Unpublished PhD thesis, School of Education and Professional Development, University of East Anglia.

Lave J and Wenger E (1991) *Situated Learning: Legitimate Peripheral Participation*. Cambridge: Cambridge University Press.

McGloin H, Adam S and Singer M (1999) Unexpected deaths and referrals to intensive care of patients on general wards. Are some cases potentially avoidable? *Journal of the Royal College of Physicians of London* **33**(3): 255–259.

McLean C, Monger E and Lally I (2005) Assessment of practice using the NHS Knowledge and Skills Framework. *Nursing in Critical Care* **10**(3): 136–142.

McQuillan P, Pilkington S, Allan A, Taylor B, Short A, Morgan G *et al.* (1998) Confidential inquiry into quality of care before admission to intensive care. *British Medical Journal* **316**: 1853–1858.

Melia K (1981) Student nurses' accounts of their work and training: a qualitative approach. Unpublished PhD thesis, University of Edinburgh.

Morgan R, Williams F and Wright M (1997) An early warning scoring system for detecting developing critical illness. *Clinical Intensive Care* **8**: 100.

Odell M, Forster A, Rudman K and Bass F (2002) The critical care outreach service and the early warning system on surgical wards. *Nursing in Critical Care* **7**(3): 132–135.

Parlett M (1969) *The Syllabus-bound Student*. Research Report. Cambridge, MA: Education Center, Massachusetts Institute of Technology.

Phillips T, Schostack J and Tyler J (2000) *Practice and Assessment in Nursing and Midwifery: Doing it for Real*. Researching Professional Education Series No 16. London: ENB.

Plowright C, O'Riordan B and Scott G (2005) The perception of ward-based nurses seconded into an outreach service. *Nursing in Critical Care* **10**(3): 143–149.

Radford M (1998) Lecture theatre. *Nursing Standard* **8**(12): 20.

Richardson A, Burnard V, Colley H and Coulter C (2004) Ward nurses' evaluation of critical care outreach. *Nursing in Critical Care* **9**(1): 28–33.

Ritzer G (1996) *The McDonaldization of Society: An Investigation into the Changing Character of Contemporary Life*, revised edn. Thousand Oaks, CA: Pine Forge.

Ritzer G (2000) *The McDonaldization of Society: New Century Edition*. Thousand Oaks, CA: Pine Forge.

Scholes J (1988) Socialisation: The Gateway to Learning. Unpublished MSc Thesis, University of Manchester.

Scholes J and Endacott R (2002) Evaluation of the effectiveness of educational preparation. *ENB Research Highlights* **49**: 1–6.

Scholes J and Endacott R (2003) The practice competency gap: challenges that impede the introduction of national competencies. *Nursing in Critical Care* **8**(2): 68–77.

Scholes J, Endacott R and Chellel A (1999) *Diversity and Complexity: A Documentary Analysis of Critical Care Nursing Education*. Research Reports Series Number 13. London: ENB.

Scholes J, Freeman F, Gray M, Wallis B, Robinson D, Matthews-Smith G and Miller C (2004) Evaluation of Nurse Education Partnerships. www.brighton.ac.uk/inam/research/projects/partnerships_report.pdf (accessed 15 January 2005).

Smart B (1999) *Resisting McDonaldization*. London: Sage.

Smith S (1988) An analysis of the phenomenon of deterioration in the critically ill. *Journal of Nursing Scholarship* **20**(1): 12–15.

Smith G, Osgood V and Crane S (2002) ALERT – a multi-professional training course in the care of the acutely ill adult patient. *Resuscitation* **52**(3): 281–286.

Stenhouse C, Coates S, Tivey M, Allsop P and Parker T (2000) Prospective evaluation of a modified early warning score to aid earlier detection of patients developing critical illness on a surgical ward. *British Journal of Anaesthesia* **84**: 663.

Trow M (1973) *Problems in the Transition from Elite to Mass Higher Education*. Berkeley, Carnegie Commission on Higher Education.

United Kingdom Central Council for Nursing, Midwifery and Health Visiting (1999) *Fitness for Practice*. London: UKCC.

Walker W (2001) Comprehensive critical care education is critical to success. *Intensive and Critical Care Nursing* **17**: 237–241.

Watson D and Bowden R (2005) *The Turtle and the Fruit Fly: New Labour and UK Higher Education 2001–2005*. Education Research Centre Occasional Paper. Brighton: ERC.

Wenger E (1998) *Communities of Practice: Learning, Meaning and Identity*. Cambridge: Cambridge University Press.

Willis J (1998) Working on expanding roles. *Nursing Times Learning Curve* **2**(9): 14–15.

Wood I, Douglas J and Priest H (2004) Education and training for acute care delivery: a needs analysis. *Nursing in Critical Care* **9**: 159–166.

Zukas M and Malcolm J (2002) Pedagogies for lifelong learning: building bridges or building walls. In Harrison R, Reeve F, Hanson A and Clarke J (eds). *Supporting Lifelong Learning, Vol. 1, Perspectives on Learning*. London: Routledge Falmer/Open University.

Chapter 6

Effecting transitions: transforming knowledge and practice

Introduction

In the previous chapter the impact of formal education on students' learning has been examined. The factors that can inhibit or promote good learning opportunities have been analysed and critiqued. Strategies to facilitate the learner's transition into the critical care environment have been proposed. In this chapter, attention now turns to facilitating practitioners, at various stages of their career, who are not on a formal learning programme.

Facilitating transitions for registered nurses

The DH in their document, *The Nursing Contribution to the Provision of Comprehensive Critical Care for Adults* (DH 2001b), identified four key stages in the clinical career for critical care practitioners:

(1) critical care assistants;
(2) registered practitioners (including critical care nurses with a specialist qualification);
(3) senior registered practitioners (critical care nurses with 4 years' experience who hold senior posts including sister/charge nurse positions, clinical nurse specialists, network leaders, practice educators and some clinical management posts);
(4) consultant practitioners.

The evolving role of critical care assistants is to be examined in Chapter 8 and this includes a critique of the issues relating to delegating competencies. The needs of four types of registered practitioner are now specifically examined. They include:

■ newcomers and novices to critical care;
■ practitioners returning to practice after a career break;

- those undertaking silent transition or 'acting up';
- inspiring horizontal transitions for practitioners who wish to consolidate their experience.

Newcomers and novices to critical care

The current recruitment and retention crisis in the NHS has been felt within intensive care units for some time (Naish, 1995; Scott, 1998; McLeod, 2001; British Association of Critical Care Nurses, 2003). Many initiatives have been set in place to improve the conditions for students or other learners in clinical environments, recognising that this will have a direct impact upon recruitment and most importantly retention (DH, 2001b; RCN, 2003; Williams *et al.*, 2003).

Critical care environments have provided D grade competency packages and in-service training as part of a robust orientation programme for almost a decade (Durston and Rance, 1995). These were in part introduced to enhance the recruitment and retention drive in response to the 'perennial staffing shortage' experienced by critical care services (McLeod, 2001). To supplement these important initiatives additional measures of support are needed to help the newcomer and novice acclimatise to the range of emotional, technical and adaptive demands of the critical care environment (Cutler, 1998). The adaptive process is highly subjective and the reactions to critical or traumatic experiences subject to personal processing and the individual's normal coping strategies (Mitchell, 1993). Therefore, formal strategies to facilitate the acquisition and assessment of competencies need to be scaffolded by moral and emotional support (see Chapter 5).

The RCN (2003) recommended that new staff joining a critical care area should have a named preceptor with whom they work for a defined supernumerary period. Two further studies examining the impact of starting out in critical care (Scholes and Smith, 1997; Kite, 1998) identified that the novice or newcomer needed continuity in working with that preceptor to help them build a rapport and trust and enable free exchange of ideas and expression of concern. In addition to the preceptor's input, working with a practice educator to support the development and assessment of their competence was an invaluable tier to facilitate and direct their learning. Clear goals of expected performance, and evaluation of how they were meeting those goals within given time frames, were important to help the individual gauge their transition and integration into the unit. Such evaluation should take account of the fact that the stress and anxiety of starting out in a new unit might initially inhibit performance with some signs of regression in practice as they accommodate new learning and technical skills into their repertoire of clinical competence (Scholes and Smith, 1997; Kite, 1998). To help newcomers and novices through this stage it was important for practitioners to feel that they were not alone. Strategies for support such as clinical supervision and action learning sets (see later in this chapter) might be useful strategies to help the individual share their experiences and find solutions to the challenges they face. In addition the appointed preceptor needs to consider specific needs of the newcomer who is a practitioner returning to practice following a career break.

The practitioner returning to nursing

One strategy to expand the staff resource has been to attract back into the service qualified nurses who had taken a career break. The most recent package to attract back returners has included financial support, although this varies from area to area. This support includes: a bursary whilst undertaking the course, no course fees, payment for the clinical placement periods of the course, help with travel costs and help with child care costs (NHS Careers, 2005). The return to nursing courses vary in length between 113 and 150 hours (nursingcourses.co.uk, 2002). They vary in content but include legislative changes in health care delivery, research and evidence-based health care, personal development, study skills, and an updating of clinical skills. Some, but not all, specifically address manual handling, the safe administration of drugs and the relevance of observations alongside an update in practical resuscitation.[1] Hours in a clinical placement are supernumerary and under the guidance of a designated mentor, and the returner can select a placement in an environment of their choosing (NHS Careers, 2005).

Returners to ICU may consider that the rapid advancement in technology, medication and treatment regimen amplifies their problems in making the transition back to practice without significant support and supervision. These nurses will have experienced a variety of life event and professional transitions that can influence their current change process. Life wisdom and people skills may compensate for the initial technological deficit in performance and could be used to great advantage by the critical care team. However, when facilitating the return of these nurses to clinical competence, account should be taken of the senior positions they might have held prior to a break in service. This can cause additional role strain where they feel that they are returning to a situation in which their knowledge and skills are made redundant by technological advances, compounded by having to slot back into a service at a status considerably lower than the one they left.

When facilitating a newcomer or novice to critical care or a return to practice nurse, it is important to demonstrate patience and empathy. Many of the ideas set out below may seem obvious, but it is because they are so 'taken for granted' that they are sometimes forgotten. This is especially the case when working through a D grade competence package or induction programme where the focus is on the acquisition of functional aspects of competence.

---

[1] These topics have been collated from a sample of Return to Nursing Course Descriptors found at www.nursingnetuk.com/return_to_nursing_cres.html?fs9001=65b299898c00c6 retrieved on 30 March 2005). In some programmes, these elements are provided by the employing Trust and are therefore not included in the course hours.

This guide is therefore set out to help the preceptor to consciously attend to the factors that will impede or enhance the learning of new skills.

Factors to consider when facilitating a newcomer, novice and return-to-nursing practitioner

The preceptee (novice or newcomer to critical care or return-to-practice nurse) may have a strong fear of failure, the implications of which extend far beyond a personal crisis and might well cause serious potential harm to the patient. This can stimulate high attentiveness and engagement in learning new things, but it might also inhibit learning and memory especially if that individual is overwhelmed with new information. The experience is exhausting. Legitimating exhaustion is important. A balance needs to be found between meeting the learning needs of the student and ensuring continuity of engagement with their preceptor, notably where 12-hour shifts are the norm within a unit.

There is a Chinese proverb which states:

> *I hear, I forget*
> *I see, I remember*
> *I do, I understand.*

Studies have shown that we remember 10% of what we hear; 25% of what we see; but 90% of what we do (Ginman, 2005). Therefore, it is essential not to overload the newcomer and novice with too much verbal information. This is difficult to measure, as normal everyday understanding and action within the critical care environment for an experienced practitioner become so integral to their way of being in the clinical world that they may either: (a) forget to articulate it; or (b) overload a newcomer or novice with complex elements of their practice without first identifying if their preceptee has a grasp of the more fundamental aspects. A framework that sets out explicit competencies and dates by which the individual is expected to achieve them will help both the preceptor to pace their induction programme and the preceptee to pace their efforts. This does not prohibit the preceptee from achieving outcomes sooner but sets realistic goals, especially in the first few days of practice.

The Chinese proverb also reminds us that demonstration, rehearsal and then consolidation are crucial to understanding. Critical care environments, by their nature, require swift and immediate interventions. It might well be very tempting, and sometimes essential, for a preceptor to make adjustments to a patient's medications, ventilation settings and other equipment and continue to do so without allowing the preceptee the opportunity to do it themselves because the avoidance of delay is essential. This is especially the case when the patient is extremely unstable or the unit is very busy. However, constant intervention or 'taking over' can undermine the preceptee's confidence and can ultimately leave all the new learning 'heard' but not practised. Empathising with the preceptee and making allowance for slow, possibly clumsy performance will ultimately be less costly in time and effort. Anxiety that slows performance which results in an intervention by the preceptor may inhibit the preceptee further, and result in them avoiding practising new skills altogether. It is therefore essential that any newcomer or novice has a supernumerary period in which they can work with someone throughout the shift to maximise opportunities for 'learning through doing' or rehearsing skills under supervision. This level of dependency on the preceptor, especially in the early days of an induction programme, should be acknowledged and allowance made to the staffing ratios throughout the unit.

Learning that is put off till tomorrow when it is timely today can extinguish 'yearning for learning', preserve the status quo and undermine confidence. Therefore, it is helpful to enable the preceptee to identify the learning that has taken place, to help them focus on where they have been effective and identify areas for further development, planning in specific learning opportunities that build upon the experience of that day. Preceptees often find returning to the same patient helps them to build their understanding in incremental steps, but they do need to be encouraged to care for a wide range of patients with different levels of dependency throughout their supernumerary period.

Another aspect that is often forgotten by the more experienced practitioner is the need to explicitly enable the preceptee to build a repertoire of language or vocabulary of critical care practice. This helps the preceptee to clearly articulate a problem that is understood by their colleagues. Relating at this level (i.e. sharing a common professional language) will also enhance the preceptee's confidence and enable them to take intellectual risks. All this requires an environment in which the individual can feel well supported and free to express any knowledge deficit, trusting in their preceptor to help them through the encounter and adjustment phase of their transition.

Scenario 6.1

A new staff nurse was working with a practice educator in intensive care. The patient to whom they had been allocated had an array of complex needs, one of which was the requirement for haemofiltration. The consultant had instructed the new nurse to increase the fluid removal rate to 80 ml. The nurse had wrongly heard this instruction and set the rate at 280 ml, not realising her error. The practice educator noticed this error after the round had left the bedside, because she was alerted to the sound of the straining rollers and pump. Intervention was made to reduce the rate back to within normal parameters without any deleterious effect on the patient. The practice educator was able to review the nurse's knowledge and explain essential aspects of safety in the management of a patient on haemofiltration.

In this example we can see how powerful language is and how this can lead to misunderstanding, especially if an individual does not have the knowledge or experience to realise their error. In this scenario, because the consultant had emphasised the need to increase the fluid drawn off quite substantially, the nurse had not thought to question 280 ml or realise he had said *to* 80 ml. This error can be seen as fundamental to anyone who has cared for a patient on haemofiltration. Without baseline experience the nurse did not know what the normal fluid removal rate was so she had no checks against which she could question the accuracy of her action. She willingly changed the setting to demonstrate to the practice educator that she had understood his explanation of the settings on the machine. Therefore, it is even more critical to reinforce in the preceptee that they question everything that they are unsure about, but in this scenario we can see that no such doubt had surfaced for the newcomer. This serves as a potent reminder to all who supervise students and new staff: knowledge is needed to ask questions. Therefore, until the new staff member has acquired sufficient insight into knowing what to ask about, when and how, they must remain under the direct supervision of an experienced critical care nurse.

Finally, throughout any induction programme regular feedback is important. The balance between positive appraisal of performance with constructive criticism and areas for further development needs to be considered. It is important to harness the positive, to identify what works well and why, and not focus solely upon error. However, in critical care there is little leeway for error and this can sometimes lead to an individual who has demonstrated fault in one area sometimes being labelled as a failure in all areas. Critical care nurses are notorious for their intolerance of the slow grasp of new skills or of performance that lacks dexterity. Some may exhibit their displeasure through non-verbal cues or sighs, and these are reported to be worse for the newcomer and novice than clear articulation of a preceptor's concerns (Scholes and Smith, 1997). All qualified staff should take some responsibility for the induction of new staff, but it is important to recognise that within a team some staff might have greater talents in facilitating newcomers or novices who are experiencing difficulty. This is not the sole province of the practice educator, although their advice and support will be invaluable.

Silent transitions: acting up

In nursing, perhaps we can consider three landmark transitions: starting our training, taking up our first staff-nurse post, and then the first sister's/charge nurse's post. These are all signified in an expression of social dress which outwardly displays the newly acquired status or position of the post-holder. However, although these landmark transitions are profoundly memorable events, subtle developmental transitions, or grade enhancements within the same unit or department can be as, if not sometimes more, stressful. This can be because there is no break with the past (ceremony of departure), no closure, no period of induction, or no outward display of changed position because rarely does the uniform or even name badge depict these changes in status. Furthermore, the expectations of the employer as to how the individual's practice should change may also go unstated. In this situation, the transitioner has to meet the expectations they have set for themselves or assume behaviours either from mirroring the substantive post-holder's performance, or from closely modelling the behaviour of others in a similar post. How realistic or ambitious the goals for performance are, the time scale for achieving them and the individual's self-appraisal of their performance will all have an impact upon the transitional process. All this has to be done in the full knowledge that they are transitioning for a temporary appointment.

It is therefore imperative within subtle career moves that the line manager and post-holder discuss their ambitions for the role and identify what might be needed to enhance performance, whether that be new skills or knowledge. If such promotion has been acquired *without* interview and or formal procedure, the post-holder should still seek the new job description and clarify the specific competencies for the post. In this way they can realistically identify what is expected of them (DiMarco, 1997). Without these the focal person has to establish their own goals and this can lead to ambiguity, unrealistic expectations and potential role strain.

An alternative approach to 'acting up' is to segment elements of one role, vacated by a prolonged absence, and divide the workload and specific responsibilities to a number of other practitioners. This can be a practical solution that has the additional dividend of staff development, but may lead to resentment and disparagement because it does not attract remuneration for the additional responsibilities. In role transition terms it may cause role strain to the post-holders who have to accommodate these additional responsibilities without the possibility of delegating tasks from their own role to others. Such a process may mask the transitional process or not even be recognised as such by either the role incumbent or role senders. Failure to acknowledge this might result in low attainment.

Such transitions are rare, but they illuminate what is often taken for granted in acquiring a new post. Many upward promotions through progression points and clinical banding, even when acquired through interview, can seem relatively subtle. Practitioners may wrongly assume that they are conferred with promotion as a result of existing performance that requires no further adjustment to fulfil all the role expectations of the new post. However, this can lead to disappointment.

The next section examines different ways of acquiring additional skills to broaden and deepen professional practice and enhance role performance.

Facilitating horizontal transitions

More recently, recruitment of newly qualified staff nurses has been less problematic, but a continuing crisis is in retaining experienced staff nurses (DH, 2000b). The challenge for these individuals and their managers is how to facilitate horizontal transitions into stimulating roles and thereby retain but also motivate nurses who may remain on the same clinical band for extended periods.

One model that has been proposed to stimulate recruitment to critical care and then retention within it is rotation programmes (RCN, 2003). Richardson *et al.* (2003) posited that these programmes can benefit all staff at whatever stage in their clinical career, including senior nurses and sisters, especially if they are to be groomed for leadership roles. However, their pilot programme started with D and E grade nurses (equivalent band 5). Their programme was established to exchange staff of equivalent grade or experience between adult and cardiac critical care units and their associated HDUs. The benefits for staff were cited as the acquisition of new clinical skills that built upon current experience, the potential for career progression, networking and fulfilling Post-registration and Practice (PREP) requirements (ibid.: 86). They surveyed all the staff involved and found that the key concern, expressed by 75% of the respondents, related to team integration in the exchange unit (because of the different shift patterns and the impossibility to exactly match clinical grade and experience); some restrictions to development opportunities and supervision (as the exchangers were not supernumerary bar the first week); and difficulties with travel arrangements (ibid.). Despite these concerns, the nurses who participated found the experience to be motivating and stimulating and that it created the opportunity to cross-fertilise ideas between units. In addition, with these new skills the nurses were then able to offer cover in times of staff sickness. However, Richardson *et al.* (2003) caution that this strategy should be a voluntary exercise, as some staff indicated that if it were made compulsory it would be sufficiently unsettling to move them to leave.

Participating in the development of new services can also stimulate and motivate staff. Services established for patient need can have the additional benefit of developing skills and enhancing relationships between the ward and unit, and stimulate critical reflection on the development team's nursing practice. Examples where these types of practice developments have had an impact, not only on service improvements but also on staff morale, include: the establishment of follow-up clinics for ICU patients run by E grade staff nurses (Strahan *et al.*, 2003: 54); nurse-led discharge from a high dependency unit (Knight, 2003); and a bereavement follow-up service (Platt, 2004). These demonstrate the direct relationship between enhancing patients' and relatives' experience of critical care services and the job satisfaction of nurses. Furthermore, it reinforces care as a core nursing value and is fundamental to patient-centred initiatives and practice developments that are mutually rewarding (McCormack and Garbett, 2000).

Funding such initiatives may become problematic if the cost per volume (or number of patients treated) is limited to care provision of level 3 patients in the intensive care unit, without any additional costs set in the tariff that acknowledges the work of outreach, or other follow-up services to provide critical care without walls (Smith, 2005).[2] However, by making explicit the

---

[2] Number of patients treated is the basis for critical care funding throughout 2005/6 but subject to critical care bed day costs being set by health resource groups in the future (Smith, 2005).

link between patient care initiatives and staff satisfaction, an argument can be made that pump priming costs for service improvements can be offset by cost savings through staff retention.

Facilitating transitions into senior posts

Developing the leadership potential in staff and promoting effective nursing leaders is seen to impact upon staff morale, motivation, retention and recruitment, professional development, quality improvements, and service efficiency and effectiveness (DH, 2001a). Networking, succession planning, shadowing, coaching and mentoring are identified as strategies to foster future empowering leaders (RCN, 2003). Importantly, the Department of Health suggests that to meet the modernisation agenda future leaders of critical care services will need to have competencies in systems working, redesign and change management (DH, 2001a: 11). However, Manley (1997) sets transformational leadership as the key skill, whereby the team work towards a shared vision or construction of possibility and that vision inspires, energises, challenges and stimulates, but it is the leader who enables others to achieve their potential based on a bond of trust.

One of the more important features to enable staff to make the transition through to senior posts is therefore an enabling leader who creates the possibilities for exploration and progress (Manley and Garbett, 2000). A second ingredient is that of critical companionship (Titchen, 1998) to facilitate the focus on transitional potential and progression through facilitated critical and supportive reflection (Elliott, 1991). In this context the practitioner is engaged in a process of making sense of an accumulation of experiences to effect transformation and emancipation (Mezirow and Associates 1990)[3].

Some authors take the position that competency-based frameworks are the antithesis of a humanistic, developmental approach to career development (e.g. Ashworth and Saxton, 1990; Elliott, 1991; Gonczi, 1994). I do not believe these two positions are mutually exclusive if the assessment of competence is taken as the baseline from which the individual builds a programme of development to effect their next transition towards expertise. I do not therefore see a competence framework for senior critical care nurses to be a contradiction in terms, if the approaches to learning for these senior posts are broad but the assessment of advanced competence is specific. However, I do not take the position that advanced competence is strictly the domain of technical roles that are exclusively designed to provide for medical substitution although such competencies would probably be easier to articulate. Some roles might

---

[3] Critical companions facilitate others through the use of observing, listening and questioning, feedback on performance, and high challenge/high support: a critical dialogue aimed at enabling the individual to articulate their craft knowledge (Titchen, 1998). The application of some of these ideas is taken up in the next chapter examining the use of assessment as a learning tool.

well incorporate areas of practice that have traditionally been the domain of medicine, but in taking up these aspects of practice the advanced practitioner brings a value-added component and a 'dose of nursing' that enhances the quality of the experience for the patient (Scholes and Vaughan, 2002). Therefore, competencies for the advanced practitioner need to capture the way in which they are able to exert their legitimate influence to improve patient care and outcomes (Ball and Cox, 2003). The same scenario can be applied to the competencies required of the consultant nurse. Most importantly for senior practitioners, they need to root out and make explicit competence embedded in their experiential wisdom. As such they may be far more holistic and broader than competencies for practitioners in earlier stages of their career.

Competencies can help the senior practitioner reflectively determine their next destination in their learning journey – either towards the expansion in their repertoire of clinical competence, or learning that enables their competent performance to be transformed into skilled craft and professional artistry (Titchen and Higgs, 2001). Clinical supervision and facilitated critical reflection are two essential tools to achieve this.

Reflection

Reflection is a process of learning whereby the individual examines their practice through an analysis of their thoughts, feelings and actions and the knowledge that went into an experience (Bulman, 2004; Johns, 2005). Reflection involves reviewing one's own values, challenging assumptions and considering broader social, political and professional issues that are relevant (Mezirow and Associates, 1990). This is important if there is to be positive social change as a result of the reflection (Atkins, 2004). Such an approach is said to evoke double loop learning (Argyris et al., 1985; Grant, 2005), but requires critical facilitated reflection if it is to be achieved (Mezirow and Associates, 1990; Atkins, 2004; Johns, 2005).

Why is reflection proposed as a tool by which an individual might self-assess their performance and promote growth and development? This might occur when an individual reaches a point of dysjuncture, whereby past routines can no longer sustain performance and an alternative solution has to be found (Jarvis, 1983). In role transitions terms, this would be when the individual is confronted by a contradiction in what they know. Eraut (1994) argues that contradiction characterises the field of experiential learning. However, as has been described thus far, an individual can defend themselves from contradiction and bury themselves in routine, and this is a recognised coping strategy for dealing with stress (Menzies, 1962).

The ultimate aim of reflection is therefore to 'trouble the mind to consider' (Johns, 2005: 150) limitations, alternative perspectives, areas for the professional to improve, areas where new information might inform practice and what part the individual practitioner has in developing the practice of themselves and others (King and Kitchener, 1994). Equally, reflection might *'raise the spirits'* of the reflectee in helping to recognise their therapeutic potential and contribution to care (Johns, 2005: 150). However, it is the former aspect which can cause a practitioner to defend themselves against deeper reflection as a coping strategy against the stress of contradiction, but that action only inhibits the process of experiential learning.

Degazon and Lunney (1995) suggest that journal writing is a powerful way to engage reflective thought that allows for the freedom of expression of feelings and perceptions without fear of exposure. Furthermore, because this can be undertaken at the reflectee's own pace and the reflectee can select their subject matter, it is in the control of the writer. However, Jasper (2003) cautions that to be an effective learning tool the journal should be completed on an incremental basis over a period of time. It should provide a record of events and experiences, and focus specifically on the learning that has occurred as a result of that experience, and contain reflective commentaries. Through this medium, reflective writing is said to develop analytical skills and critical thinking; foster creativity; engage the writer in examining new perspectives and knowledge; and demonstrate how much we understand and the limitations of our understanding (Jasper, 2004).[4]

In this way the learning journal is a powerful tool for personal development and self-empowerment (Moon, 2000). Profiles built as a result of such writings have been advocated as a means by which expert practitioners might be accredited (RCN, 2002). Furthermore, such a strategy is advocated as a means of realising advanced practice because it can capture the knowledge of the art of nursing which is embedded in the practitioner's performance but is rarely articulated in the literature (Fulbrook, 2004). However, to sustain this level of engagement with a journal requires high levels of motivation. Building profiles towards accreditation is one mechanism to get the process started but it can only be sustained if found to be personally fulfilling. Such an approach does not, however, suit everyone's learning style (Miller *et al.*, 1994) and in these cases interactive processes to facilitate reflection can be more effective.

Strategies for facilitating interactive reflection

Clinical supervision

Facilitated, purposeful reflection on clinical issues is usually referred to as 'clinical supervision'. Much of the discussion about clinical supervision has focused upon the activity in mental health nursing, counselling, psychotherapy and social work, and it is a relatively new concept within acute

---

[4] It is these higher order notions of analytical skills and critical thinking that often link reflective writing with postgraduate accreditation of higher levels of practice. Although reflective writing, particularly in portfolios, is a common approach to practice assessment in most programmes, including pre-registration courses, the level of sophistication in the reflective writing should be relative to the stage of the professional maturity of the learner (Endacott *et al.*, 2004).

and emergency care (Maddison, 2004). However, the lack of robust empirical studies to establish the relationship between reflection and clinical supervision in the reflectee/supervisee (Bulman, 2004), and more importantly the ultimate impact this has on the quality of patient interactions (Grant, 2005), render much of the theoretical discourse about the topic rhetorical polemics. Advocates claim that experience demonstrates the value of the approach (Bulman, 2004) and that it can guard against burnout, reduce sickness rates and increase staff morale (Butterworth *et al.*, 1997).[5] However, other studies have illustrated significant barriers to the successful introduction and maintenance of high quality supervision (Duncan-Grant, 2001). This may account for why the adoption of clinical supervision is patchy and inconsistent (Maddison, 2004). Despite these reservations, the value of the process itself is considered to be extremely powerful, although the organisational forces which can hamper clinical supervision might be more powerful (Duncan-Grant, 2001). Despite these reservations, clinical supervision has been proposed as a means to assure the safe delivery of patient care (UKCC, 1996)[6] although latterly this has shifted to the assessment of competence (DH, 2000a, 2001a; National Audit Commission, 2001).

In clinical supervision an 'expert' facilitates a colleague to examine a piece of work or clinical practice and asks the following questions (Borton, 1970). What was happening and why? What was done or said and how was that handled? Could it have been handled differently to enhance outcomes; if so, how? Therefore, the approach to clinical supervision is reflective analysis of a clinical situation, rather than the specific assessment or judgement by another of the performance of the person being assessed (Spencer *et al.*, 2000). This is important as many suspect clinical supervision to be some form of duplicitous quasi-counselling that doubles as organisational surveillance. O'Riordan (2002) points out that it is entirely inappropriate for supervisors to act as therapists. However, Bodley (1992), in an analysis of the distinction between counselling and clinical supervision, found that there was indeed overlap between the two processes and that it was essential to have a skilled supervisor to work within those grey areas. This is particularly the case when a supervisor is acting as a professional coach to facilitate the transition of the supervisee, and in critical care where the emotional aspects of practice need to be addressed. There is, however, a distinction between facilitation and therapy:

---

[5] Butterworth *et al.* (1997) undertook evaluation of clinical supervision in 23 nursing and mental health sites. This study has been seriously criticised because: (a) individuals who took part had no training in clinical supervision and demonstrated that they had diverse interpretations of the practice; (b) the measures presupposed the benefits of clinical supervision to be those of reducing staff sickness and burnout and improving staff morale and; (c) the researchers set out to prove that CS worked and paid no attention to the potential Hawthorne effect the experiment might have created in the first instance (Duncan-Grant, 2001).

[6] The concept of clinical supervision first advocated by the Department of Health's *Vision for the Future* (DH, 1993).

both may deploy similar strategies to enable the expression of concern and discovery of solutions, but therapy focuses on the personal and clinical supervision on the professional. However, as has already been stated, life event transitions can impact upon professional transitions. The clinical supervisor might help their supervisee to draw on past successful coping strategies to help them through their current transition, whereas a therapist might work more extensively on enabling the individual to find new ways of coping and being in the world that include the review of the causes of psychological fragility. Bodley (1992) suggested that a contract negotiated between the supervisor and supervisee would help to make explicit the boundaries of the supervisory process. This indicates that prior to the successful introduction of clinical supervision there needs to be careful planning, clarification of intent and preparation of staff.

Factors to consider when introducing clinical supervision to critical care

First, there needs to be a commitment to critical facilitated reflection expressed by the organisation, supervisor and supervisee. That means they 'walk the talk' and deliver: clinical supervision is not considered a luxury but a sacrosanct activity that is recognised as a core component of clinical governance (Grant, 2005).

Secondly, it is essential that supervisors and supervisees receive appropriate training. The assumption that someone who is senior can automatically do this is faulty (Platzer, 2004). Furthermore, organisations can wrongly assume that trained staff need longer workshops than untrained staff, and supervisors need longer workshops than supervisees (Grant, 2005: 13).

Preparatory workshops for supervisors need to enable the acquisition of (Carroll, 1996):

- attentive skills to be alert to the learning needs of supervisees, focusing on different aspects of work with patients;
- tracking skills to probe and pursue critical reflective analysis on aspects of practice;
- ability to recognise when to intervene and when to hold back;
- cooling-out strategies to help close the supervisory sessions;
- evaluative strategies to establish the learning that has taken place from clinical supervision;
- procedure/policy for managing disclosures that indicate that the welfare of patients or the supervisee might be at risk.

Supervisees, on the other hand need preparation to help them plan for the supervisory session including (Carroll, 1996):

- selecting what to present in supervision;
- deciding how to process their learning within clinical supervision;
- knowing how to evaluate the learning that has taken place from the supervisory session and how to transfer this learning back to patient care.

Table 6.1 Factors inhibiting the implementation of clinical supervision (CS).

Proctor's 1986 model cited by Butterworth and Faugier (1992)	Duncan-Grant's critique (2001)
Formative/educative	CS as an act of avoidance ■ Supervisor fails to check assumptions, or to evaluate the learning that has taken place – supervisee defending themselves from examining potential contradictory learning experiences. ■ Unwillingness of supervisee and supervisor to engage in critical reflection as both committed to non-reflective task orientation.
Restorative/supportive	CS as 'time out' ■ Distinction between a 'cosy chat and a cup of tea' accompanied by 'outpouring of their tales of woe' and something that challenges and builds on practice. ■ Refusal to process, remember or focus on unwanted memories from practice. ■ Supervisor's reluctance/lack of confidence to probe the complex or emotionally laden aspects of practice.
Normative/managerial ■ quality assurance tool ■ organisational selling point ■ individual audit of corporate work practice	CS as act of collusion ■ Public expression of support undermined in practice, e.g. service provision comes before clinical supervision – so practice remains unscrutinised. ■ CS disrupted – phone calls, knocks on door, bleeps. ■ Supervisee selective about what they raise in CS to defend self and organisation from critique.

Finally, to be effective, the supervisor and supervisee need to ensure that the sessions are purposeful and educative. Some of the factors that might inhibit the successful delivery of clinical supervision are illustrated in Table 6.1.

Group facilitation offers an alternative approach to address some of these issues.

Group supervision

Grant (2005) advocates the use of public peer supervision. In this the supervisee and supervisor go through the process before a group who observe their practice and then take part in the supervisory discussion. In this way, teams can effectively engage in purposeful deliberation about issues, learn the skills of effective supervision, and deal with attitudes, feelings and values. The extent to which this exercise would result in 'managed or staged' presentation of the issues would rely on the advanced skills of the supervisor and absolute confidence and trust in those who observe the event. However, such an approach helps to focus the team's attention on the educative purpose of the session. It would help to avoid personal projection of issues on to others (blame culture), and to focus the work on critical reflection rather than 'a cup of tea and a whinge' session. It would also serve to demonstrate that these sessions are not about personal counselling. When topics of a more personal nature are to be raised, or when failing performance is in question, alternative strategies for support should be used.

Clinical supervision has been promoted as an approach to facilitate stress management through the analysis of critical incidents (Cotterill-Walker, 2000). However, it might be that the process of critical reflection on issues that create stress might heighten anxiety as they are brought into the foreground of people's attention before successful strategies are adopted to reduce the impact of stressors (O'Riordan, 2002). Therefore, if these issues are to be managed in a group setting, the facilitator should be alert to an individual's need for debriefing following the session.

Critical incident analysis and incident trails

Critical incident analysis can be managed through case reviews or incident trails. These tend to be factual examinations of events and analysis of patient data that influenced clinical judgement rather than an examination of feelings, behaviours and attitudes that surrounded the event. A whole team approach to the analysis can serve to amplify potential learning from others. They are useful to help identify the sequence of events, tighten protocols and satisfy all those concerned that an incident has not passed without scrutiny.

Fineman (1993, 2003) talks about the way in which organisations manage emotions and how certain areas within buildings are designated for the display of particular emotions, for example the coffee room, the office, the teaching room, the kitchen, the relatives' lounge, the changing room. These are recognised zones where emotional behaviour is distinct from that on the clinical floor. However, permission for specific emotional expression is also dictated by who is present within those locations at the time. Therefore, incident analysis by the clinical team, facilitated by a harassed consultant, in a teaching room heavily attended by doctors in training, and restricted by time limitations, all serve to manage the event and steer away from an examination of feelings. The absence of coffee and cake, when it is custom and practice to have them at the meeting, might serve to indicate the seriousness with which the matter is being viewed. Such practice serves to bring to the foreground unwanted memories of events, but these will remain unresolved in a meeting of this type. Furthermore, there is a risk that critical incident analyses focus entirely on errors, and create negative emotions that inhibit rather than inspire learning from the experience. Once again, attention to the need for individual debriefing following these sessions is critical.

Action learning sets

Action learning sets (McGill and Beaty, 1995) are groups that are brought together with a common aim, that of problem solving. Members of the group may not be doing the same thing but have a common interest, for example a group of nurse consultants who meet regularly to present issues relative to the challenges they face in implementing their new role.[7] Each member of the group is given an uninterrupted period of time in which they present to their peers who actively attend to what is being said. Members of the action learning set then pose questions to enable the individual to think more deeply about the issue and make implicit assumptions about their practice explicit. The purpose is not to provide advice, although useful points of reference might be shared with one another. Support is provided in the form of a question, which helps the individual to examine the issue from an alternative perspective that can surface contradiction and potential conflict (Johns, 1999). Silences are powerful indicators of time in reflection (Platzer, 2004). However tempting it might be to rescue someone from the discomfort of such an experience, the group should attempt not to intervene, allowing the speaker to resume their response once they have assembled their thoughts (McGill and Beaty, 1995). Through this process the individual is empowered to find their own solutions to the challenges they face.

Initially a group may feel safer with an experienced facilitator. However, as the group matures, it will self-manage the time allotments and equity in attention (McGill and Beaty, 1995). The sets need to take place in an environment of trust and support (Platzer, 2004) which does not allow for interruptions that might disrupt the concentration of the group so mutually agreed ground rules are an essential starting point for the group. Bleeps therefore need to be left with a colleague.

Conclusion

This chapter has examined a range of strategies to enable critical care practitioners to grow and develop throughout their careers. All the strategies cited in this chapter are independent of formal educational programmes, but could be used for work-based accreditation of learning. However, their primary purpose is to engage practitioners in experiential learning. These experiences

---

[7] Action learning sets are particularly helpful to a group who are sharing a similar experience: for example, a cohort of newcomers, novices and return-to-practice nurses; a cluster of people who are each leading service improvements or practice developments; a group of practitioners establishing new roles within the Trust; or a group of managers leading innovation and change. They are commonly used in postgraduate educational programmes to support students through their research. Whatever the group, some element of commonality is important to ensure that the individual can then speak of the challenges they confront to an empathic audience.

might ultimately result in the individual recognising that it is time to embrace new challenges and upward mobility, but, equally of importance, they can stimulate and motivate horizontal transitions towards greater professional satisfaction and role development to enhance patient care.

All these strategies have been presented to help the critical care nurse to identify areas of strength in their performance and build upon weaker aspects to explicitly guide them on their journey towards expertise. In critical care practice there are specific aspects of a role where patient safety demands that there be explicit judgement on the individual's capacity to function competently. Therefore it is crucial to state that strategies aimed at self-learning can only scaffold quality assurance or peer assessment of the individual's knowledge and performance in practice. The next chapter goes on to address strategies of assessment to assure progression and, when identified, how to manage poor performance.

References

Argyris C, Putman R and Smith D (1985) *Action Science*. San Francisco: Jossey Bass.

Ashworth P and Saxton J (1990) On 'competence'. *Journal of Further and Higher Education* **14**(2): 3–25.

Atkins S (2004) Developing underlying skills in the move towards reflective practice. In Bulman C and Schutz S (eds). *Reflective Practice in Nursing*, 3rd edn. Oxford: Blackwells: 25–46.

Ball C and Cox C (2003) Part One: Restoring patients to health – outcomes and indicators of advanced nursing practice in adult critical care. *International Journal of Nursing Practice* **9**: 356–367.

Bodley D (1992) Clinical supervision in psychiatric nursing: using the process record. *Nurse Education Today* **12**: 148–155.

Borton (1970) *Reach, Touch and Teach*. London: McGraw Hill.

British Association of Critical Care Nurses (BACCN) (2003) Position statement on the role of health care assistants who are involved in direct patient care activities within critical care areas. *Nursing in Critical Care* **8**(1): 3–12.

Bulman C (2004) An introduction to reflection. In Bulman C and Schutz S (eds). *Reflective Practice in Nursing*, 3rd edn. Oxford: Blackwells: 1–20.

Butterworth T and Faugier J (1992) *Clinical Supervision and Mentoring in Nursing*. London: Chapman & Hall.

Butterworth T, Carson J, White E, Jeacock J, Clements A and Bishop V (1997) *It is Good to Talk'. An Evaluation Study in England and Scotland*. Manchester: School of Nursing, Midwifery and Health Visiting, Manchester University.

Carroll M (1996) *Counselling, Supervision. Theory, Skills and Practice*. London: Cassell.

Cotterill-Walker S (2000) Debriefing in the intensive care unit: a personal experience of critical incident stress. *Nursing in Critical Care* **5**: 82–86.

Cutler L (1998) Do intensive care nurses grieve for their patients? *Nursing in Critical Care* **3**: 190–196.

Degazon C and Lunney M (1995) Clinical journal: a tool to foster critical thinking for advanced levels of competence. *Clinical Nurse Specialist* **9**: 270–274.

Department of Health (1993) *A Vision for the Future*. Report of the Chief Nursing Officer. London: HMSO.

Department of Health (2000a) *The NHS Plan: a Plan for Investment, a Plan for Reform* (available at//www.doh.gov.uk/nhsplan/nhsplan.htm).

Department of Health (2000b) *Comprehensive Critical Care: A Review of Adult Critical Care Services*. London: DH.

Department of Health (2001a) *Working Together, Learning Together, A framework for life-long learning for the NHS*. London: DH.

Department of Health (2001b) *The Nursing Contribution to the Provision of Comprehensive Critical Care: a Review of Adult Critical Care Services*. London: HMSO.

DiMarco C (1997) *Career Transitions. A Journey of Survival and Growth*. Scottsdale, Arizona: Gorsuch Scarisbrick.

Duncan-Grant A (2001) *Clinical Supervision Activity among Mental Health Nurses: A Critical Organizational Ethnography*. Portsmouth: Nursing Praxis International.

Durston M and Rance A (1995) Bridging the theory–practice gap in the ITU with in-service education. *Intensive Care Nursing* **11**: 233–236.

Elliott J (1991) Competency based training and the education of the professions: is a happy marriage possible? In Elliott J (ed.). *Action Research for Educational Change*. Milton Keynes: Open University Press: 118–134.

Endacott R, Gray M, Jasper M, McMullan M, Miller C, Scholes J and Webb C (2004) Using portfolios in the assessment of learning and competence: the impact of four models. *Nurse Education in Practice* **4**(4): 250–257.

Eraut M (1994) *Developing Professional Knowledge and Competence*. London: Falmer Press.

Fineman S (1993) Organizations as emotional arenas. In: Fineman S. (ed.). *Emotion in Organizations*. London: Sage.

Fineman S (2003) *Understanding Emotion at Work*. London: Sage.

Fulbrook P (2004) Realizing advanced nursing practice through reflection. *Nursing in Critical Care* **9**: 255–256.

Ginman K (2005) *Be Your Own Confidence Coach. Easy Techniques to Achieve Ultimate Self-confidence*. London: New Holland Publishers.

Gonczi A (1994) Competence based assessment in the professions in Australia. *Assessment in Education* **1**(1): 27–44.

Grant A (2005) Supervisor practice and evaluation within an organisational context (e document). University of Derby, on behalf of the Global University Alliance (www.gua.com).

Jarvis P (1983) *Professional Education*. London: Croom Helm.

Jasper M (2003) *Beginning Reflective Practice*. Cheltenham: Nelson Thornes.

Jasper M (2004) Using journals and reflective diaries within reflective practice. In Bulman C and Schutz S (eds). *Reflective Practice in Nursing*, 3rd edn. Oxford: Blackwells: 94–112.

Johns C (1999) Reflection as empowerment? *Nursing Inquiry* **6**: 214–249.

Johns C (2005) Reflection on the relationship between technology and caring. *Nursing in Critical Care* **10**(3): 150–155.

King P and Kitchener K (1994) *Developing Reflective Judgement: Understanding and Promoting Intellectual Growth and Critical Thinking Skills in Adolescents and Adults*. San Francisco: Jossey Bass.

Kite K (1998) Learning to doubt: the professional development of nurses in one intensive therapy unit. Unpublished PhD Thesis, University of East Anglia.

Knight G (2003) Nurse-led discharge from high dependency unit. *Nursing in Critical Care* **8**: 56–67.

Maddison C (2004) Supporting practitioners in the process of reflective practice. In Bulman C and Schutz S (eds). *Reflective Practice in Nursing*, 3rd edn. Oxford: Blackwells: 73–93.

Manley K (1997) A conceptual framework for advanced practice: an action research project operationalising an advanced practitioner/consultant nurse role. *Journal of Clinical Nursing* **6**: 179–190.

Manley K and Garbett R (2000) Paying Peter and Paul: reconciling concepts of expertise with competency for a clinical career structure. *Journal of Clinical Nursing* **9**: 347–359.

McCormack B and Garbett R (2000) *Concept Analysis of Practice Development*. Executive Summary. London: RCN.

McGill I and Beaty L (1995) *Action Learning: a Guide for Professional, Management and Educational Development*. London: Kogan Page.

McLeod A (2001) Critical care assistants: from concept to reality. *Nursing in Critical Care* **6**(4): 175–181.

Menzies I (1962) Nurses under stress. *International Nursing Review* **7**: 9–16.

Mezirow J and Associates (1990) *Fostering Critical Reflection in Adulthood. A Guide to Transformative and Emancipatory Learning*. San Francisco: Jossey Bass.

Miller C, Thomlinson A and Jones M (1994) *Learning Styles and Facilitating Reflection*. English National Board for Nursing, Midwifery and Health Visiting Researching Professional Education Series 2. London: ENB.

Mitchell J (1993) Comprehensive traumatic stress management in the emergency department. *Emergency Nurse Association Monograph Series* **1**: 3–13.

Moon J (2000) *Reflection in Learning and Professional Development. Theory and Practice*. London: Kogan Page.

Naish J (1995) Recruitment crisis returns. *Nursing Management* **1**: 6–7.

National Audit Commission (2001) *Hidden Talents: Education, Training and Development of Healthcare Staff in the NHS Trusts*. London: Audit Commission.

National Health Service Careers (2005) FAQ, Working in the NHS. NHS careers. www.nhscareers.nhs.uk/nhs/cb_faqs.html (accessed on 30 March 2005).

Nursingcourses.co.uk (2002) You want to return to nursing . . . . nursingcourses.co.uk/Flowchart/fcy4y.html (accessed 30 March 2005).

O'Riordan B (2002) Why nurses choose not to undertake clinical supervision – the findings from one ICU. *Nursing in Critical Care* **7**: 59–66.

Platt J (2004) The planning, organising and delivery of a memorial service in critical care. *Nursing in Critical Care* **9**: 222–229.

Platzer H (2004) Are you sitting comfortably? From group resistance to group reflection in several uneasy steps. In Bulman C and Schutz S (eds). *Reflective Practice in Nursing*, 3rd edn. Oxford: Blackwells: 113–127.

Richardson A, Douglas M, Shuttler R and Hagland M (2003) Critical care staff rotation: outcomes of a survey and pilot study. *Nursing in Critical Care* **8**: 84–89.

Royal College of Nursing (2002) *Expertise In Practice Project (Pilot)*. London: RCN Institute.

Royal College of Nursing (2003) *Guidance for Nurses Staffing in Critical Care*. London: RCN.

Scholes J and Smith M (1997) *Starting Afresh: the Impact of the Critical Care Milieu on Newcomers and Novices*. ITU NDU Occasional Paper Series Number 1 (University of Brighton) [ISBN 1 87 196692 2].

Scholes J and Vaughan B (2002) Cross-boundary working: implications for the multi-professional team. *Journal of Clinical Nursing* **11**: 399–408.

Scott H (1998) Government launches new recruitment campaign. *British Journal of Nursing* 7: 304.

Smith C (2005) Meeting unmet need: the challenge ahead. Editorial. *Nursing in Critical Care* **10**(4): 165–166.

Spencer M, Kinnear K and Vieira D (2000) Clinical supervision: a challenge for critical care nurses. *Nursing in Critical Care* **5**(3): 142–146.

Strahan E, McCormick J, Uprichard E, Nixon S and Lavery G (2003) Immediate follow up after ICU discharge: establishment of a service and initial experiences. *Nursing in Critical Care* **8**: 49–55.

Titchen A (1998) *A Conceptual Framework for Facilitating Learning in Clinical Practice*. Occasional Paper Number 2, Centre for Professional Education Advancement, Lidcombe, Australia.

Titchen A and Higgs J (2001) A dynamic framework for the enhancement of health professional practice in an uncertain world: the practice–knowledge interface. In Higgs J and Titchen A (eds). *Practice Knowledge and Expertise in the Health Professions*. Oxford: Butterworth Heinemann.

United Kingdom Central Council for Nursing, Midwifery and Health Visiting (1996) *Position Statement on Clinical Supervision for Nursing and Health Visiting*. London: UKCC.

Williams S, Coombs M and Lattimer V (2003) *Workforce Planning for Critical Care: A Rapid Review of the Literature (1990–2003)*. Southampton: Faculty of Medicine, School of Nursing and Medicine, Southampton University (available from www.modern.nhs.uk/criticalcare).

Chapter 7
Assessment as learning

Introduction

This chapter will examine the way in which assessment can be used as a learning tool to facilitate transitions and enable progression through to expertise. The argument is made that assessment can be viewed as a starting point rather than an endpoint and that, when assessment is couched in these terms, it is the catalyst to ignite further potential. As such, assessment is seen as a critical component to facilitate development through constructive challenge and therefore a model that has currency throughout the practitioner's clinical career.

One of the key issues in developing expertise is to identify weak performance and seek to turn this round. Achieving excellence and expertise does require individuals whose performance is significantly substandard to be weeded out from the profession. In critical care, this is even more essential because of the scientific knowledge and technical knowhow that inform clinical judgement and clinical practice. In short this affects patient safety. A weaker capability to function with compassion and thoughtfulness is equally important but often harder to objectify and act upon. Nevertheless, to achieve expertise, both scientific knowledge and professional artistry are needed. If an individual, through assessment, can identify areas for further development, this can trigger the contradiction that can ultimately transform their performance. This is why assessment is presented as a tool for learning.

Assessment is a critical component of professional self-regulation and is essential to maintain public trust and confidence in the profession (Asbridge, 2003). To take action when weak performance is identified is often painful and uncomfortable. Handling such situations might require the assessor to develop a new set of skills and competencies. Indeed, some may become an expert in assessment, although basic assessment skills are an essential component within the repertoire of any nurse so she might notice substandard performance, take action to support and remedy that, and, where necessary, take action to fail a student who is unable to achieve an appropriate standard.

The first part of the chapter deals with the unpalatable notion of failing students and why the concept of failure to fail has become such a hotly debated issue. Many of the approaches and strategies examined can be used to work alongside a colleague whose practice has raised some concern. This may be even more uncomfortable, but an assessor is reminded that, ultimately, enabling someone to see that they will not be able to achieve, effects an important transition for them: leaving the profession and finding more suitable employment. Although extremely stressful to take such action, it can be a powerful learning experience for the assessor, acting as a catalyst to confirm their core values and standards of nursing practice.

The chapter then moves on to address strategies for using assessment to help people to achieve good practice. It may be the first time that a practitioner has been confronted with the contradiction that their performance is not considered adequate. Therefore, the assessor requires skills to enable that individual to revisit, refresh, reconstruct and revise their approach, ultimately leading to a significant adaptive transition and enabling them to start out on their journey to achieve their potential.

Failing to fail

Studies since 1990 (e.g. Lankshear, 1990) have identified a problem with mentors and assessors being reluctant to fail students. Recent studies have identified that this is a prevalent and current problem (Watson and Harris, 1999; Norman *et al.*, 2002; Duffy, 2003; Scholes *et al.*, 2004), with a distinct inconsistency in the number of students who fail practice relative to theoretical assessments (Duffy, 2003; Scholes *et al.*, 2004).

The factors causing this are varied, with some common concerns in the reluctance to fail pre- and post-registered students. However, there are some subtle distinctions between the reticence to identify failing colleagues (who may be post-registration students on clinical programmes, but may be colleagues undertaking competency assessment) and the failure to fail students on pre-registration courses. The factors can be broadly categorised under three headings:

- procedural;
- differing agendas of academic and clinical communities;
- the validity and reliability of the practice assessment documentation.

Procedural issues

To fail a student is procedurally and emotionally difficult (Duffy, 2003). The time it takes to collate information and make a case for failure or referral is disproportionate to the time it takes to give the student the 'benefit of the doubt' and pass them (ibid.). Set against other immediate clinical priorities, making the decision to fail a student is not taken lightly. However, where the practice assessment procedure enables a student to carry forward certain aspects of their clinical work to be assessed in another setting, assessors are more likely to make a decision not to decide, providing a rationale that the student has had inadequate experience or consolidation of skills during that placement (Scholes *et al.*, 2004). Summative points in the assessment procedure force the issue, but decisions to fail a student are only taken when performance is seen to be distinctively faulty. This is because mentors feel that the course of action they must take sets them up to be judged by their peers, their managers and the academic staff in the university (Lankshear, 1990; Hrobsky and Kersbergen, 2002). As such, failing a student is seen to be an 'act of courage' by the mentors even though this is recognised as a component of their professional responsibility (Duffy, 2003).

Confidence to fail a student is critical. This requires the mentor to be sure of their decision and the course of action they must take, and secure in the knowledge they have adequate evidence to support their decision. The requirement to report concerns early can be problematic, as the assessor may find objective evidence to support their concern hard to pin down at that stage (Hrobsky and Kersbergen, 2002). This can be made more difficult when there has been a lack of continuity in working alongside the student, and/or no insight into their clinical performance up to that point (Duffy, 2003; Scholes *et al.*, 2004). Therefore, borderline performance can be offset by allowances made for the clinical specialism of the placement, difficulties settling into new teams, or the progression point of the programme. In these situations, students are invariably 'given the benefit of the doubt' (Duffy, 2003). However, allowances made at the outset may serve to undermine the assessor's case later in the procedure. Therefore, mentors require time to be allotted to supporting weak students, making explicit their concerns, and clearly identifying the action taken to help the student retrieve the situation (Hrobsky and Kersbergen, 2002). Managers may not always be in a position to dedicate time for a mentor to do this. However, failure to follow the process to the letter can result in the decision being over-ruled by the higher education institution (HEI) through the appeals procedure (Duffy, 2003; Scholes *et al.*, 2004). Such a threat fundamentally contributes to the problem of 'putting pen to paper' (Duffy, 2003) and starting this uncomfortable course of action.

This task may be made more complex when educational jargon (Duffy, 2003) and complex educational taxonomies to illustrate progression and academic levels of performance may obfuscate the aspects of practice to be assessed (Scholes *et al.*, 2004). As a result students may reach the end of their programme without having practised a range of fundamental or advanced skills (ibid.). In addition, competencies written to a level of abstraction to enable their application to a range of clinical settings may prove to be too loose to provide reliable triggers for mentors to identify weak or failing performance. In such a scenario, the student may achieve some aspects of a learning outcome adequately, but certain elements may not be attained to the mentor's satisfaction. Once again, this may give rise to mentors erring towards the positive, especially when a mentor is prepared to take a student's personal circumstances into account to militate against failure (Duffy, 2003). Importantly, when assessors find the assessment tool vague, they may respond by writing obscure comments which do not help to specify the weaknesses in students' performance. Therefore, students are not provided with clear, explicit goals to redress the shortfall and can continue to migrate through their clinical placements with only a vague idea that there is a problem. This is particularly challenging when an assessor's primary concern is the student's lack of insight into their own performance (Scholes and Albarran, 2005).

Tools that lacked specificity to capture students' professional attitude, behaviour, presentation of self, or punctuality have been found to have frustrated mentors (Scholes *et al.*, 2004). Academic staff were perturbed that mentors were unable to make the links to outcomes, which they felt could capture such deficits in performance if they applied lateral thinking. However, mentors were seeking explicit statements against which they could provide concrete examples to identify points of failure, whereas academic staff were attempting to broaden the areas of students' performance to be assessed. However, this left some mentors feeling unsafe because their task was to provide a water-tight case to uphold a decision of failure but the documentation seemed too vague to make this clear cut. For these reasons many mentors considered that failing the students in practice should be the school's job[1] (Duffy, 2003).

Scenario 7.1a: Warning signs – 'attitude problem'

Stephen, a third-year pre-registration student, had been allocated to the coronary care unit for his critical care placement. On arrival he made known to his assessor, Sarah, that he was there to learn how to read ECGs. When Sarah explored if he had any other learning goals for the placement, Stephen presented his skills book, stating he needed to get these 'ticked off'. Although it was half-way through the third year, hardly any of the third-year skills had been signed off by mentors. Sarah accepted Stephen's defence that he had not given this priority due to meeting the deadlines for a series of academic assignments. In the first week of the allocation, Sarah noticed that Stephen spent much of his time at the nurse's station

---

[1] In some HEIs, an assessment process had been created whereby the academic staff did pass or fail the students' practice assessment. The mentors' role in this case was to verify the evidence provided by the students to support their competence. This decision had been made because their moderation procedures for assessment could not be realistically accommodated in the practice setting (Gerrish *et al.*, 1997). To provide academic credits for practice, which constituted 50% of the course, practice assessment had to be presented in a written format that could be reviewed by moderators and upheld by the exam board. In this situation, practitioners were concerned about what was being assessed: the students' written or clinical skills. An alternative approach adopted by a number of HEIs was to give the power to mentors to pass or fail a student's clinical performance, but a module could only be accredited if the student passed practice (ibid.).

reading books or talking with members of the health care team. When asked to blanket bath a seriously ill patient, he refused, stating that he was not here to be used as a 'pair of hands'. He had 'spent too much time doing personal care, running around, making beds and he wasn't allocated to critical care to do that'.

Sarah noticed that he frequently requested to leave practice to study in the library, or leave early in the afternoon to ensure he could safeguard his 'reflective time'. When challenged, Stephen complained that he wasn't learning anything on the placement. Sarah therefore arranged to work directly with Stephen the next day and to go through some of the clinical skills book. To her dismay, the next day Stephen phoned in sick. Sarah was then due for her days off, and was on night duty when she returned a week later. Stephen was on study days and had changed his off duty to work on opposite shifts, claiming he had family commitments which could not be broken. Sarah asked her colleagues to carefully monitor Stephen's performance, but no one individual had worked directly with him throughout the allocation. In the final week of the allocation Sarah managed to rearrange the off duty to work alongside Stephen. She found him careless in his clinical care and noticed he regularly made offhand remarks to other staff and made inappropriate comments to the patients. Sarah decided that Stephen's performance was inadequate and she had to refer his practice assessment.

Stephen was extremely angry about this outcome and vowed he would appeal against her decision, claiming inadequate supervision, failure to identify and support suitable learning situations, and a personality clash with Sarah. Much later, Sarah heard that the student's appeal had been upheld by the university and that he had gone on to finish his training.

In this scenario the student presents a number of triggers to alert the mentor to potential problems. These include a significant attitude problem, lack of enthusiasm about nursing, an over-emphasis on book learning and the acquisition of technical skills, and avoidance of direct contact with both patients and his mentor (Hrobsky and Kersbergen, 2002). In this scenario, Sarah used these triggers to alert her to be extra vigilant and watchful over the student (Rittman and Osburn, 1995). Furthermore, she attempted to work directly with Stephen to give him an opportunity to demonstrate his skills or illuminate areas where further development was required. However, she did not take formal action at this stage by clearly stating her concerns to Stephen, nor did she devise a clear written action plan to pass on to her colleagues. In part this was because she took into account Stephen's personal circumstances (Duffy, 2003).

Some mentors feel that to fail someone is vindictive and harsh and contrary to the professional core construct of caring (Duke, 1996). Therefore, they feel it is kinder not to fail or make clear issues of concern, especially in the early stages of an allocation (Duffy, 2003). If a student seems to be particularly defensive, a mentor may find the situation more problematic or anxiety provoking, fearing the consequences for team morale or creating a situation whereby they set themselves up for personal criticism (Lankshear, 1990). However, rigid thinking, lack of personal insight, and defensiveness to feedback were personality traits identified in occupational therapy students (OTs) who failed clinical assessments (Gutman *et al.*, 1998). Furthermore, in this ten-year retrospective analysis of failing student records, it was found that the failed OTs were unable to learn from their mistakes, and 95% of them externalized responsibility for mistakes to their supervisors, the patients, or academic situation (ibid.). If Sarah had been equipped with this knowledge, would she have felt more confident to take the bold step and take formal action sooner? Probably not, without significant support, advice and feedback from her colleagues, managers and academic staff (Hrobsky and Kersbergen, 2002).

Scenario 7.1b: The consequences of inaction

Sarah attempted to collate more information by working directly with Stephen. When he phoned in sick, she suspected this had been done as a measure to avoid direct supervision of his clinical performance. However, she felt unable to use this example to support her case without evidence that Stephen had not been genuinely unwell. Fragmented contact meant that time passed and direct supervision could not be arranged until the final week of the placement. The student's appeal was upheld on the grounds that the student was not given adequate notice of his failing performance at a stage when he could be supported through to success.

Sarah felt betrayed by the lecturing staff and her colleagues and subsequently refused to mentor pre-registration students. In addition, colleagues on the coronary care unit concluded that the emotional anguish and time taken for the referral procedure was not worthwhile as the university systems favoured the student, resulting in the mentor being judged rather than the student.

Differing agendas

The latter part of this scenario demonstrates a distinct difference between the academic's apparent response to the clinical assessor's decision and what Sarah might have expected to happen. The academics fostered a facilitative approach to retrieve the fail, whilst Sarah, who had already taken remedial action, concluded that the student should be removed from direct patient care (Lankshear, 1990; Rittman and Osburn, 1995). Therefore, where a mentor had made an assessment of a student's performance and found that the student had been placed in an alternative environment (from the universities' perspective, retrieving the fail), the mentor saw this as criticism of her mentoring skills and judgement (Hrobsky and Kersbergen, 2002). Furthermore, research has shown that a number of clinicians (and academics) were concerned that financial penalties invoked once attrition rates rose above 13% favoured the student's case if the practice failure went to appeal (Scholes *et al.*, 2004a).

The appeals process has created other anomalies. For example, conduct that would be the basis for discontinuation on professional grounds might not be recognised as a reason for dismissal from the university (Duffy, 2003). Therefore, a student might be discontinued for plagiarism, but not for theft of a patient's property if the client decided not to press charges (Scholes *et al.*, 2004a). The Council for Heads and Deans debated this issue. It was concluded that the situation was too complex to issue national guidelines, but emphasised the importance of establishing clear local guidelines in order to ensure that this anomaly might be rectified (Turner, 2005). However, the evaluation of the *Making a Difference* (MAD) curriculum concluded that: 'fundamentally, expanding student numbers and curbing attrition whilst retaining the quality of the practitioners who register was considered unsustainable' (Scholes *et al.*, 2004a), and that 'a certain level of attrition should be considered a quality marker, especially where students are discontinued through failure to meet standards in practice' (ibid.).

The students' perspective

Students gave greater priority to academic assignments as they saw these to be a greater threat to their progress than practice assessments (Scholes *et al.*, 2004a). Where they had clinical competencies to fulfil, there was a tendency for them to tick these off and move on to the next set, rather then revisit or consolidate these skills later in the programme unless specifically required (ibid.). This was because the assessment load was considered too great to take on additional challenges. Furthermore, students found that with this assessment load they needed to prioritise as they attempted to balance work–life pressures and carry out additional work to supplement their income (ibid.).

Recent studies on attrition have identified the following stressors (Magnussen and Amundson, 2003: 262):

(1) difficulty balancing home and college demands;
(2) time pressure;
(3) financial concerns;
(4) feelings of distance from faculty and staff in the clinical setting;
(5) stress associated with feeling unprepared for clinical practice;
(6) feeling incompetent in clinical skills.

In addition, it was found that where students were exposed to mentors who were unwelcoming and demonstrated a lack of basic civil discourse and manners, in combination with other problems, this could be the final deciding factor to leave nursing (Scholes *et al.*, 2004a).

Scenario 7.2: Red Flag – 'high support'

Samantha arrived in A&E on the first day of her critical care placement. She was particularly anxious about the experience, having watched a number of TV dramas and documentaries. She felt unprepared to cope with the severity of illness and range of clinical experiences she might encounter. She was also anxious about how she might 'fit in', assuming the personality and approach to nursing held by staff in A&E would differ significantly from her assumptions about caring.

Samantha is a single parent. She could not afford child care for her daughter, but within her cohort of students she found a number of other single parents in a similar situation and they had decided to form a supportive group who took it in turns to care for the children. Therefore, each morning she had to drop off her daughter at the home of the parent taking care of the children that day. Sometimes this would require a complicated journey on the public transport system before she set off to the hospital. Therefore, to arrive on time for an early shift, she would have to set the alarm for 5.30 am.

Samantha had struggled with her academic assignments. She found it particularly difficult to create clear time to attend to her essays and complete her portfolio. She constantly felt pressure to meet the competing demands of the course and find sufficient time for her daughter. She resolved this by working late into the night. By the third year of her course she was suffering from extreme fatigue. A sleepless night worrying about her first day in A&E had exacerbated her exhaustion.

When she arrived she was directed by a harassed receptionist to the staff room. There she found a number of students looking equally lost. The practice educator for the department was due to spend the day with the students introducing them to the unit and talking about meeting their learning needs. Due to a sudden bereavement, the practice educator had been given compassionate leave. Unprepared for this eventuality, it was decided that four students would be sent home to undertake personal study, whilst the remainder would work alongside the qualified staff in the department. Samantha elected to stay as she had child cover that day.

Samantha was allocated to work alongside Paula, a staff nurse with four years' clinical experience in A&E. Paula had resisted undertaking her mentorship course, understanding from colleagues that the local programme was 'rubbish'. She took a fairly dim view of students and the local HEI provider, considering the quality of the students to be poor and the preparation of the students for A&E deficient.

She noticed that Samantha appeared extremely anxious and tired. When she asked her why she looked so 'terrible'. Samantha explained her situation. Paula stated that she thought the arrangements made for child care could contravene the law because the students did not have a licence as child minders. She stated that they were 'particularly hot on child protection in A&E and she should be very careful'. Later in the day Paula made known to Samantha her views on the quality of training at the university and also made some extremely derogatory comments about the nursing profession. She told her to 'keep up and pay attention' or get out of the way if something 'went off' which she felt she could not manage.

Samantha felt unclear as to how to respond to these remarks. She assumed that she should give Paula as much space as possible, fearing she might further alienate or anger her. Samantha hovered at the desk responding to her instructions, which became more truncated and directive as the day progressed. Anxiety and exhaustion got the better of Samantha, who retreated to the staff room in tears. Paula discovered her ten minutes later and barked: 'Go home! You are no use to us here'. She then phoned the college to advise them of what had happened and to make a complaint about Samantha.

The dynamics in this scenario make clear how a student may perceive her reception to be unwelcoming. Experiences throughout the day compounded rather than refuted Samantha's anxieties. Exhaustion and nerves led her to a course of action which set her up for further criticism. However, Paula's unsympathetic stance and concern to meet the needs of the department obscured her attention to Samantha's situation. The central issue in this scenario is: what course of action would be the best one to take to revise this situation? One helpful strategy is to ask the student to perform clinical skills that might be expected of a more junior nurse to provide opportunities for her to demonstrate success and build confidence (Rittman and Osburn, 1995). However, due to the novelty of work in A&E and the student's heightened state of anxiety, it might have been more fruitful to allow the student to closely observe the mentor that day and undertake aspects of care once they had been demonstrated and Samantha's competence to do them had been assured (Scholes, 1998). In part the mentor attempted to do this but conveyed this in a confusing instruction to 'keep up and pay attention' or 'get out of the way if something went off which she couldn't manage'. In this situation the use of colloquial subcultural phrases did no more than to accentuate Samantha's outsider status. This was extremely unfortunate as her needs were for acceptance and inclusion, and the role strain she experienced resulted in further alienation and criticism. There were mitigating circumstances within the department to make allowances for some of the things that happened, but Paula's distinctly curt response to Samantha obscured them.

Why do we find the circumstances from scenario 7.1 to be different from the circumstances in scenario 7.2? How could these differences be perceived by the mentors (role senders) and how did they fundamentally influence the mentors' reactions to the situation and subsequent action? Table 7.1 outlines some of the distinctions in the messages sent out by the students and how these were interpreted and acted upon by the mentors.

Of note is the vulnerability of Samantha's situation relative to the defensive position taken by Stephen. Samantha demonstrates high commitment, motivation and struggle against considerably difficult circumstances and this lends us to be sympathetic and supportive of her position. Self-disclosure has enabled the reader to take far more of her personal circumstances into account when

Table 7.1   Comparison of student and mentor responses using role transition theory.

Moderators	Stephen	Samantha
Personality	Defended, rigid thinker, poor comportment with colleagues and patients	Highly motivated, anxious to succeed
Attributional style	Blaming others: lack of supervision, no learning opportunities, personality clash	Self-blaming, defers personal needs in favour of others
Locus of control	Internally contained	Projected externally – significant inter-role conflict – work–life balance out of control
Self-esteem	High	Low
Confidence	High	Low – self-doubt dented by exhaustion, anxiety and fear about being unable to respond to patient need
Social identity	Technical, academic nurse	Single parent – student nurse
Social network	Weak within the group	Single parent support group, student cohort
Centrality of role to self	Poor – contested identity as a nurse	High, income and independence hinged on success on course
Emotional reactions	Anger	Anxiety and exhaustion
Cognitive reactions	Reinterpreting events, redeploying attention to academic and technical learning	Confirmation of all anxieties and assessment of dissonance in values of caring

making a judgement about her performance. However, Stephen's approach is confrontational; his over-confident manner, assertiveness of position and demand for specific learning are not matched by a willingness for his performance to be reviewed or by a commitment to complete work set out in the assessment documentation. Therefore, one suspects Stephen's motivation and commitment as a nurse.

The two students were subject to quite distinct approaches from the mentors. Samantha's mentor was unsympathetic, forthright and unsupportive, preying upon her vulnerability rather than reacting and supporting her through her anxiety and exhaustion. In contrast, Stephen's mentor gave him the benefit of the doubt and fostered a stance of high challenge, high support and genuine concern to enable him to progress. One wonders what would have happened if Samantha and Stephen, by some extraordinary twist of fate, had been allocated to the alternative placement.

The validity and reliability of the practice assessment documentation

The validity and reliability of assessment documentation have been found by Norman *et al.* (2002) to be wanting. These authors based their conclusions on a survey of seven Scottish HEIs which examined how the clinical competence of student nurses and midwives was assessed. In this context 'reliability' refers to the situation whereby the outcome stated in the practice assessment document is consistently assessed irrespective of context and circumstances, and 'validity' refers to the reality of what has been assessed. Norman *et al.* (2002) concluded that no single method was appropriate for assessing clinical competence. However, clearly stated competencies, with specific criteria for performance, are more likely to reflect the reality of critical care practice and to consistently focus the assessor's attention on what is to be specifically assessed than are broad or abstract learning outcomes (Scholes and Endacott, 2002).

The language used to describe learning outcomes or competencies can be too broad to specifically locate certain skills (Scholes *et al.*, 1999). As a consequence, students can reach the end of their programme without being assessed in some key areas. Many academics were concerned about the quality process that practice assessment was supposed to ensure, especially in being able to make confident recommendations that the student was fit for the register at the end of the programme (Duffy, 2003). Therefore, it is critical for the students (and their mentors) that what is to be assessed and what is expected of both parties are made transparent (Rhodes and Tallantyre, 1999). To resolve this problem, explicit skills schedules or competency statements have been introduced to help focus the assessors' attention (Scholes and Endacott, 2002; Scholes *et al.*, 2004). However, even where skills lists have been compiled, research findings indicate that these can be unreliable (Scholes *et al.*, 2004). The following scenario was drawn from the evaluation of nurse education partnerships (ibid.).

Scenario 7.3:   The OSCE assessment

In one HEI, the academic staff began to doubt the validity and reliability of the practice assessment process. In response to these concerns they established an Observed Simulated Clinical Examination (OSCE) in the skills laboratory so they might directly observe student performance in specific skills including lifting and handling, and the taking and recording of blood pressure. This examination was set for the last module in the first year of the branch programme, two years after the students had started this course. In the formative assessment, only four out of a cohort of 120 students passed the OSCE. The shocked academics reviewed all the students' practice assessment documentation, in particular the skills schedule, and found all the students had a mentor's signature against the skill 'accurately record physiological parameters', implying that they had performed this to the assessor's satisfaction in practice. This was particularly troubling as the lecturers, who were acting as the patients in the OSCE, were concerned that many students had made up the findings, rather than documenting accurately what they had heard. The lecturers knew their normal resting blood pressure and therefore any wide deviation from this led them to be suspicious of the students' competence, especially where there was wide variation between the students' recordings. Their concerns were heightened when three students applied the cuff to the lower arm, one allegedly around the neck of a lecturer (standing in as a patient) and one student put their ear to the patient's arm to listen for a blood pressure. Although some leeway was given for the anxiety created by the OSCE, there was profound disturbance among the academic and clinical community that such a finding could be possible among second-year adult branch students, especially as all of them had been in acute clinical areas on a number of occasions, routinely recording patients' physiological parameters.

The advocates of the OSCE were pleased that the examination had identified this weakness, and enabled intensive remedial interventions to be set up to reverse the apparent level of incompetence. However, at the summative assessment just under 60% of the cohort passed and it was feared that this assessment was so discriminatory it would have to be dropped as the university could not tolerate this high level of failure in their attrition figures.

Brown (1999) suggests that reliable and verifiable evidence of competence is best collected from multiple sources which triangulate to support any claim made by the student. However, explicit, relevant criteria need to be stated to ensure that this approach is effective. In the scenario above, the triangulation of evidence between the skills schedule and OSCE proved that either performance was highly variable in the skills laboratory relative to the clinical environment, or that the standards for the assessment of practice were substantially different between the tutors and the mentors (Brown, 1999: 104). Although this example serves as a stark reminder of the disparity and lack of equivalence that might occur between mentors and tutors, it also highlights the lack of validity and reliability of practice assessment documents to locate and prioritise what needs to be assessed and how.

Some practice assessment documents explicitly identify what types of evidence are required to establish competence, i.e. what must be directly observed and what might be determined through other media, for example question and answer, testimonies, product evidence (project, case study, video, tape recording, reflective accounts, product or literature search), by demonstrating, by inference, that the learning outcomes have been attained (Rhodes and Tallantyre, 1999). However, within a skills schedule, the intention for practice to be observed is implicit, but may not be explicitly stated. When skills schedules have been designed to shift their assessment from a training model to an educative one, other forms of data can be used to illustrate the learning that has taken place to inform the performance of that skill. However, these forms of data can take precedence over direct observation, especially where the mentor assumes the student's competence by default, i.e. that faulty performance has not been brought to the mentor's attention on this placement, and they can assume competence because the student has progressed to this point having been assessed by others before them. Where practice is seen to be so 'everyday', fundamental skills may go unobserved in favour of evidence that demonstrates the advancement of a core skill or knowledge. This example serves as a timely reminder that no such assumptions can safely be made, and a mentor has to assure themselves that the student is indeed competent in the 'basics'. The safest method to do this is through direct observation or through probing questions. This is essential for anyone new to critical care where the environment might inhibit the student, newcomer or novice from applying their fundamental caring skills, or where attention to the application of more basic knowledge may be avoided in deference to the attention they feel they need to pay to the technology and machinery that support the patient (Scholes and Smith, 1997).

Questioning

The key challenge for mentors and assessors is making explicit certain aspects of practice through questioning. Returning back to the basics and exploring the fundamentals of care, patient assessment, technology management and so forth, can be bypassed on the assumption this has been done before. Indeed, students may find it extremely challenging to describe what is 'normal'. In critical care the use of physiological and biochemical parameters may serve this purpose, but establishing a descriptive language for normality as seen, heard, felt, smelt or touched in a patient assessment can prove to be very illuminating to establish baseline comprehension of anatomy and physiology. Further exploration of 'feelings' about a patient, in terms of severity of illness or mood, can be a useful starting point to get the student to consider the data on which they are basing their assumptions.

Posing questions that are 'reasonable' or 'at the right level' to gauge the knowledge and understanding of the assessed can prove to be challenging. Coping with this can be achieved through the process of probing questions which explore both the breadth and increasing depth of understanding. Thus as one question is answered, this leads on to another issue for exploration, often following a trajectory of increasingly complex or critical situations. Ultimately this can end with exploring the student's understanding of concepts abstracted from the concrete situation which stimulated the questions in the first instance, and can examine their application to different clinical situations. This type of lateral thinking and questioning unfolds as a dialogue. Plumbing the depths

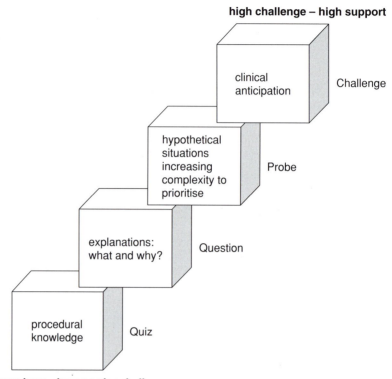

high challenge – high support

clinical anticipation — Challenge

hypothetical situations increasing complexity to prioritise — Probe

explanations: what and why? — Question

procedural knowledge — Quiz

functional know how – lower order challenge

Fig. 7.1 The hierarchy of questions.

of a student's knowledge in this way can be very rewarding, but it does take time and considerable confidence and the student has to trust their assessor for this to be effective. However, what this achieves is an exploration of the student's ability to be flexible and adaptable and most importantly to anticipate events in practice. The model in Fig. 7.1 demonstrates the hierarchical set of questions that can be used by assessors to assess the student's level of understanding and thinking in action.

Scenario 7.4: Questioning to identify competence

A student was met by their personal tutor to discuss their learning experiences on the surgical HDU. The student said that her mentor was off sick and that she was working alongside an agency staff nurse. She had been allocated to a patient who had gone for a long and complex operation, and although she had been offered the opportunity to follow the patient into theatres to observe the procedure, the student had declined as it was estimated to take up to six hours. The tutor asked about the planned operation. The student told her that it was: 'the reversal of an ileostomy and formation of a colostomy'.

This seemed a strange procedure and the tutor pursued the point with the student. The student checked her handwritten notes from the handover and confidently restated that the operation was 'the reversal of an ileostomy and formation of a colostomy'. The tutor then asked her why she was having the reversal of an ileostomy, to which the student replied 'because she (the patient) doesn't like it'. The tutor then attempted to get the student to recognise this was unusual because the ileum was proximal to the colon and therefore, if the stoma was to be formed as high as the ileum, this was because the colon was diseased. If temporary, then the ileostomy was likely to be reversed because the colon had sufficiently recovered, but the formation of a second stoma in the colon would be extremely unlikely. The student was adamant that this had been reported in handover and did not seem to follow the tutor's reasoning (assuming the tutor was not aware of current practice). So they checked the patient's notes and found the patient was having a *colectomy* and *reformation of an ileostomy* due to progressive bowel disease.

The tutor realised that the student's underlying knowledge of anatomy and physiology was deficient. This left the student with insufficient knowledge to recognise the 'strangeness' of the operation as she had described it. The fact that none of the trained staff had challenged this as strange at report left the student feeling vindicated for her silence. However, this lack of knowledge alerted the tutor that she needed to check the student's understanding of how to care for the patient following this operation.

At that point the patient returned from theatre. The tutor suggested that they should go to the patient and receive the handover and go through the physical assessment and checks that would need to be undertaken to assure the patient's safe post-operative monitoring. The student stated that she would prefer to keep going through the theory in the office, and the agency nurse 'would be able to do the obs'.

In this scenario, quizzing the student about the patient's operation revealed unconscious incompetence. Using the model of question and answer to probe the student's level of understanding and then integration of new information, the tutor attempted to address the deficits in performance. The attempt here is to ensure a minimum standard of safety for the patient. The approach taken has been outlined to provide an illustration of how the hierarchy of questions (see Table 7.2) can be used to enable the student to identify and remedy deficits in knowledge and clinical competence.

This is a very simple and basic list that would need to be completed to ensure that the student was safe to continue to care for that patient in the immediate post-operative period. The tutor took the option to undertake a full physical assessment of the patient with the student, so they might go through all these aspects, tying in the knowledge with activities of care. In this way, it was hoped that the student could memorise this learning and attach this to visual cues within the physical assessment process. This does not have to be detailed,

Table 7.2   Example of the hierarchy of questions.

Procedural knowledge
- What observations would you record and why?
- Ensure student understands and can competently perform recording of pulse, blood pressure, CVP measurement and urine output, and monitor output from the nasogastric tube.
- Ensure student knows how to recognise a healthy stoma stump and to report any deviation from the norm. Ensure the student knows how to monitor the wound dressing for signs of excessive oozing or blood loss. Ensure the student knows how to monitor wound drains to ensure they are patent and functioning, and give guidance about how much loss would be expected and when to report abnormal loss to the nurse in charge.
- Ensure the student understands the fluid replacement regime, and setting the rate of the pump.
- Ensure the student understands the pain management regime and when to review this if it does not control the patient's pain.
- Ensure the patient's nausea is managed and there are strategies for keeping the patient comfortable.
- Have all aspects been covered? If not, plug the gap with further cues; where dangerous levels of misunderstanding are evident, provide immediate information as to what to do and why.

Questions
- What is the meaning of these data?
- Assess student's understanding of signs of hypovolaemic shock, neurogenic shock and sepsis.
- Ensure the student understands signs of fluid overload.
- Have all aspects been covered? If not, plug the gap with further cues; where dangerous levels of misunderstanding are evident, provide immediate information as to what to do and why.

Probing
- Given the procedure lasted for six hours, what other potential complications do you need to monitor for?
- See if the student recognises the risks of pressure damage, hypothermia and post-operative reactions to anaesthesia, and how to assess for these.

Clinical anticipation
- Check to see if the student is aware of longer term complications associated with the surgery.
- Assess to see if the student is aware of signs of sepsis; if she recognises the basic stages of psychological adaptation the patient might well go through; and understands the social implications of this surgery.

Closure
- Ask the student to identify the two things they have learnt from that experience. From each one of those items, get them to identify two aspects of learning that they need to follow up in personal study. Critically, assure the student that this will be followed up and their new knowledge evaluated in subsequent interaction in clinical practice. This level of engagement is likely to motivate the student and assure them that their learning will be evaluated.

but is done to seek assurance of a safe level of understanding. It may seem time consuming, but a mentor would only need to do this on one occasion to assure themselves that the student could be safely entrusted with that patient's care. The longer term consequences of failing to do this could be far more time consuming, and potentially hazardous for the student and her mentor but more importantly for the patient.

In some situations where such deficits in knowledge were identified, practice educators might be called upon to help facilitate the process of handling weak or failing students, especially where service pressures placed additional demands on the staff nurse (Watson and Harris, 1999).

The practice educators

To support the major revision to the pre-registration programme initiated by *Fitness for Practice* (UKCC, 1999) and the recommendations of *Making a Difference* (DH, 1999), a new role was introduced: the practice educator. Their role was to increase the capacity and quality of learning environments and to support mentors with supporting students. In part, their role was to help mentors understand the practice assessment documentation and facilitate greater understanding of the procedures necessary to support weak or failing students. Some of the activities in which they engaged to support mentors included:

- developing specific examples of experience available in different settings to match the learning outcomes;
- making practice assessment documentation more accessible;
- building mentor confidence in undertaking rigorous assessment of student competence;
- working with mentors to accurately record the outcomes of their interventions so that documentation could be presented to the appropriate assessment board;
- working directly with students in practice and establishing developmental packages and learning contracts;
- undertaking summative practice assessment of students;
- feedback intelligence to the college about areas of practice development and potential new learning environments, thus spreading the student load among a wider pool of potential mentors.

In addition they assumed an arbitration role which included some of the following activities:

- deciphering the practice assessment book for students and mentors;
- resolving disputes between students and mentors, notably around delays in completing learning outcomes or lack of interest in the students;
- offering advice on how to handle personality clashes;

- writing to an awards board outlining exceptional circumstances and providing evidence to support a claim for an exceptional third attempt in their practice assessment;
- assuming a pastoral role to support students with personal difficulties (Scholes *et al.*, 2004).

As such, the practice educators have proved to be an invaluable resource in helping mentors to address aspects of handling problematic students. Therefore, if a mentor does encounter difficulties with a student, it is strongly recommended that they seek the counsel of someone who assumes such a post or its equivalent.

Assessment of post-registered students

A significant issue for assessing students on post-registration courses is that they are colleagues. Therefore, to formulate a judgement on the performance of a 'student' when they are a clinical colleague the next day heightens the vulnerable position of the assessor and the potential consequences for the individual being assessed. Solutions to this problem might be either to assume that the student was competent to get on the course in the first instance or to assume the student is competent in their everyday practice and that what is to be assessed is the acquisition of new or advanced skills (Endacott *et al.*, 2003). Another strategy might be to select an assessor who can objectively view the student's performance, either because of their relative seniority to the student or by virtue of their position within the clinical team, or appoint multiple assessors (Scholes and Endacott, 2002). However, the latter found that performance had to be significantly below par to invoke a refer because to take such action could significantly increase the paperwork and might create tensions within the clinical team.

Critically, assessment of colleagues tended to take place away from the bedside and followed a more reflective and discursive examination of the issues. In many instances, students and mentors identified that assessment took place outside the clinical setting. This was because they considered their role to be about 'filling in the documentation' rather than assessing the individual student. Further, this approach was often taken by highly committed mentors and students because they wanted to dedicate time to the activity, which, if done in work hours, could be subject to service distractions. However, under these circumstances, it made it particularly problematic for the assessor to highlight deficits in performance (Scholes and Endacott, 2002).

As has been indicated, performance had to be significantly below par to be noticed by an assessor. When this is extended to noticing weak performance in colleagues who are not on a formal taught programme, the problem can be even greater. Up to this point the assessment of learners on formal education programmes has been addressed. The next section of the chapter addresses peer evaluation of colleagues.

Transforming the practice of demotivated colleagues

The first stage in noticing weak performance may be an assessor's emotional reaction or 'gut instinct' about the practitioner (Burkitt *et al.*, 2001). The assessor may have initially picked out patterns of behaviour and clear visual cues which seemed too imprecise to be expressed. For example, this may be in the individual's body language or in their interaction with others (ibid.). This is described by Rolfe (1997) as 'fuzzy logic' whereby the assessor has applied certain 'rules' of expected behaviour to the assessment of their colleague but the deficits in performance seem too vague to pin down, and/or the assessor feels too unfocused for them to be acted upon. This might initially dissuade the assessor from taking further action. However, with careful consideration, the assessor can distil objective evidence from the weak performance to make explicit what needs to be addressed. In this situation the assessor may find that they have to work backwards from their initial conclusion and then work through the reasons for the initial 'hunch'. This may leave some assessors uncomfortable with the process, as it seems that they are deliberately seeking negative examples to exemplify their case when in fact they are seeking evidence to either refute or confirm their initial suspicions. Furthermore, if an assessor considered that such an approach is often taken to the formulation of clinical decisions, they might feel less anxious about the process.

Table 7.3 highlights some cues which might alert a qualified nurse of poor performance in colleagues at various stages in their clinical career.

Once these signs of weak performance have been identified, it is important to take a series of steps to redress the shortfall and give the individual the opportunity to turn their practice around. This can be done in various stages of intervention. The steps below identify interventions at various stages to facilitate the transitions necessary to restore and then maintain a highly reflective, critically evaluative, professional performance. They are:

- recognition of one's own limitations;
- confronting contradiction and creating high intellectual interference;
- critical self-reflection.

Step 1: Recognition of one's limitations

It is critical for the assessor to enable the individual to recognise their limitations and take responsibility for their own learning (Rhodes and Tallantyre, 1999). To do this, they will need to have their performance deficit made explicit so they might recognise how others see them.

Wherever possible, aspects of good performance need to be identified as well as bad, using the format of the 'critical sandwich'. However, some assessors avoid the critical filling, and fail to get to the point of their evaluation. Therefore, a prepared case with examples of poor performance should be presented to the individual, and this gives them something concrete to focus

Table 7.3   Noticing poor performance.

Newcomers to ITU
- Focus on sequencing tasks – inability to multitask or reflexively manage situations as they arise.
- Alarms flashing and the nurse not responding to these – resulting in a series of other alarms being triggered in quick succession; slow response to these alarms as the nurse attempts to work out how to resolve the situation.
- Standing back and slowly processing information, inability to read chunks of information and react to the situation.
- Excessive time planning and problem solving but responses tend to be reactive and few are made proactively.
- Predisposition to focus on menial tasks.
- Excessive time spent on the computer reviewing patient data.
- Time spent away from the patient.
- Observations late, drugs administered late.
- Inadequate information conveyed at report or to the ward round.
- Poorly prepared for ward round – information not readily available.
- A disorganised bed space, patient does not appear to be left comfortable.

D grade staff nurse < 6 months in post
- Superficially looks to be managing with observations recorded on time, patient looks comfortable, time management seems to be adequate.
- Recognises and can prepare information that would normally be requested at ward round or handover. However, inability to cope with anything other than 'routine', and when questioned demonstrates a superficial understanding and a lack of insight into interpreting the data.
- No risk taking, no proactive decisions.

D grade staff nurse > 6 months in post
- Will follow procedures but reluctant to progress the patient, preferring to maintain stability rather than move the patient on to the next stage.
- Waiting to be led, needs to be questioned as a catalyst to get them to take the next step or be bolder.
- Needs directive cues to help them to make connections between different sources of data.
- May avoid contact and/or defend against direct supervision to avoid exposing their superficial awareness.
- Strategy is to maintain the appearance of being 'cool', having 'things under control' and maintaining the status quo.

Senior D grade nurse
- Learnt repertoire of responses to situations but unable to provide a more complicated account when challenged at anything more than a superficial level, i.e.
  - inability to read trajectories and proactively intervene;
  - inability to make connections between different sources of data and give a sound rationale for decisive action or inaction;
  - inability to recognise individual patient responses or patterns of behaviour in response to care interventions.
- Pigeonholes information and unable to concept translate or use past experience to inform care planning.
- Reluctant to unpick a situation and analyse alternative approaches to care.
- Not challenging or capable of constructive criticism of colleagues.

Table 7.3 (cont'd)

E grade
- Regresses back to performance expected of D grade.
- Completes necessary tasks but then sits with back to the patient.
- Lacks motivation or commitment to supervise or support junior colleagues.
- Does not participate within the team or take on any additional responsibilities.
- Withdrawn, lack of motivation, low self-esteem, dip in confidence.
- Perception of hitting a glass ceiling with few opportunities for promotion so withdraws interest from within the clinical team and invests greater interest in personal life or work outside the unit.
- Reluctance to seek promotion as it is seen as more hassle.
- Financial remuneration given priority over professional progression.

F grade
- Limits activity to shift leading and maintaining the status quo.
- Unprepared to challenge and address weak performance in others.
- May have unlimited boundaries with the rest of the clinical team – junior staff may take liberties and relax standards (cardigans and coffee on the unit).
- Climate of *laissez faire*, basics or routines addressed but not proactive or dynamic in leadership and practice development.
- Relatives waiting outside with nurses sitting at the desk.

G grade
- Loss of vision.
- Loss of focus on team issues and leadership.
- Poor team management.
- Focusing on administrative tasks, sickness returns, off duty or paperwork.
- No imagination to lead practice developments, inspire the uptake of new roles, support staff to gain wider experiences, or progress the team.
- Failure to engage in the wider hospital community.
- Self-limit the amount of work they will do.

Each one of these situations can spark a regression back to former level of performance and below

---

upon and helps them to reflect on an appropriate action plan. From this point, the assessor and individual practitioner can negotiate practice experiences for more successful performance, confidence building and incremental development towards the desired standard of practice. Some hypothetical concerns that might alert an assessor to take action are illustrated in Table 7.4. This is not an exclusive list, but one that starts to unpack common areas of concern.

Once identified the individual will require a transparent and reliable system for action planning, reviewing progress and arranging further assessment of their progress (Rhodes and Tallantyre, 1999). The relationship of trust and mutual respect is critical between the assessor and the assessed to enable progression and development from the identified deficits in performance (Phillips *et al.*, 2000).

The use of explicit competences, with clear performance criteria, is helpful in determining knowledge or technical skills deficits (Jeffrey, 2000). They clearly distinguish operational competence rather than academic competence (Barnett,

Table 7.4 The triggers to notice poor performance.

Triggers	Sources of evidence
Attitude – behaviour ■ *Laissez faire* attitude in practice, insufficient effort, lack of interest ■ Weaker effort relative to other students in the environment ■ Defends against situations of direct challenge and observation of performance ■ Positions self in alternative environments away from direct observation and questioning	■ Minimal evidence to support competencies; portfolio poorly constructed and incomplete ■ Poor engagement with mentors, participation in seminars, teaching sessions ■ Excessive deployment of visits and association with advanced and technical procedures
Missed communication ■ Missed information, failure to report relevant information to appropriate personnel, inability to be proactive	■ Teaching reports, ward rounds and handovers
Missed aspects of care ■ Apparent discomfort of the patient ■ Aspects of care omitted or late ■ Drugs administered late ■ General condition of the bed space ■ Slow response to alarms ■ Actions deferred unnecessarily	■ Watchful vigilance, standing back and noticing how the student managed their workload – noticing if the individual is unable to keep on top of rapid change in a patient's condition

1997). The outcome is unambiguous when the individual is declared either competent or incompetent on the day of assessment. However, by breaking down elements of performance into component parts so they might be assessed, other critical elements of nursing practice can be missed (Rushforth and Ireland, 1997). At the basic level of assessment, and to assure patient safety, this might be the starting point, or ultimately the end point if performance gives rise to serious concern (Milligan, 1998). The required knowledge as well as indicators for successful performance need to be clearly stated to enhance the validity and reliability of the tool (Eraut, 1994), but also to serve as a clear template for any remedial action plan.

Step 2: Confronting contradiction creating high intellectual interference

To enable reflective personal insight into areas of weakness, the individual needs to be able to handle the contradiction of being confronted with feedback that suggests performance is not adequate. The first stage is to enable the individual to own the deficit in their performance. This can be achieved by using strategies that create high intellectual interference or exposure to new knowledge which renders past performance or knowledge inadequate. Figure 7.2

high intellectual interference

- higher order Q & A of 'hot' event
- critical reflection of 'cool' event
- student-triggered teaching
- teaching reports

- direct observation with real time Q&A
- nurse-led ward rounds
- amnesty: revisiting skills
- reviewing notes, x-rays, meds, obs

office/pseudo clinical ———————————————— **clinically situated**

- ward-based teaching sessions
- assignments
- student-triggered Q&A
- book learning – non-applied

- novel skills teaching
- non-reflective independent practice

low intellectual interference

Fig. 7.2 Transforming the potential: high intellectual interference model through question and answer techniques (reproduced from Scholes and Endacott, 2002 with permission of the NMC).

compares strategies which invoke high intellectual interference, and these have been compared with less directive strategies which may potentially defend the individual from critical self-reflection.

As can be seen, the factors have been divided between learning opportunities that are created in the clinical setting and those in the office or pseudo-clinical setting. The aspects that create the highest potential for contradiction occur when the individual is exposed to new knowledge relating to their current clinical practice, rather than exposure to learning which surrounds new skills or is initiated by the student. This is because, where new or advanced skills are to be acquired or where the student can self-limit or manage their exposure to new learning, they can defend themselves from significant contradiction and therefore high intellectual challenge which might trigger a significant transformative development (as summarised in Fig. 7.3). It might be that episodic exposure to low intellectual interference can build into a transformative contradiction, but this does require the individual to be sufficiently insightful to recognise this.

Although this model was developed from analysing student's clinical learning on the former ENB critical care courses, the strategies identified can be used to help a practitioner whose performance is below par to recognise and take action to remedy any shortfall in their performance. Furthermore, the more ingrained this approach becomes within the culture of the organisation or unit, the greater the norm for peer- and self-assessment, which makes it far more likely to be tolerated and viewed as less stigmatic (Jordan, 1999). Indeed testament to this fact is how staff will tolerate exposure to critical reviews of their performance when this is conducted by a trusted and respected practice educator. This is because the practice educator may be seen to be an expert in assessment and have greater knowledge of standards, and thereby can apply rules of parity and equivalence when assessing. As the practice educator role makes them slightly marginal to the core clinical team, critical review can create less disturbance to overall team morale. However, the practice educator

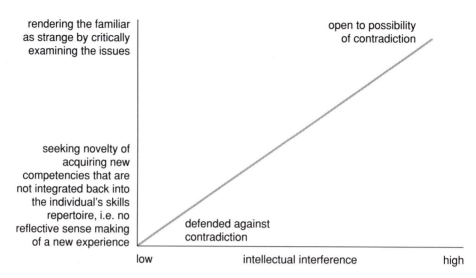

Fig. 7.3 Low and high intellectual interference in familiar and unfamiliar situations.

requires their own nexus for support and forum for discussing issues, and this is most helpful either within the critical care management team or with other practice educators and academics (Phillips *et al.*, 2000).

A comprehensive although not exhaustive set of learning activities have been set out by the Northern Ireland Practice and Education Council for Nursing and Midwifery, NIPEC (2004). These have been identified in Table 7.5 and clustered into triggers which might engender significant learning opportunities that evoke high intellectual interference. Each one of the items identified will only stimulate high intellectual interference and potential for transformative learning if the individual practitioner is prepared to render the familiar as strange, make sense of the situation through critical facilitated reflection, and be open to the possibility of contradiction or new learning which is then integrated back into the professional repertoire of the practitioner. Learning through such an approach is crucial to enable a practitioner to make the journey towards expertise.

Step 3: Critical reflection and self-evaluation

Assessment as a learning tool is grounded within an iterative process whereby initial assessment inspires critical self-reflection and new learning which is then assessed (Brew, 1999). However, Mezirow and Associates (1990: 7) remind us that: 'thoughtful action is reflexive, but is not the same as acting reflectively to critically examine the justification of one's beliefs'. Genuine capture of new learning and how this sits within the existing repertoire of professional knowledge and the art of nursing therefore comes out of purposeful reflection (Titchen and Higgs, 2001).

Table 7.5 Identifying learning opportunities, assessment and feedback strategies to promote high intellectual interference (NIPEC, 2004).

Learning from the workplace	Self-directed activity	Formal learning strategy
Supervised practice Q&A (hierarchy of questions)	Posing knowledgeable questions	Learning contracts Assessment tool Competency framework
Buddying	Peer review	Mentoring junior colleagues
Coaching	Follow-up learning in response to reflective triggers	Evidence of reflective account submitted for evaluative feedback
Critical reflective facilitation	Reflective diary	Clinical supervision Critical incident analysis
Research groups/journal review club/seminars	Preparation of presentation to group Critical appraisal of research	Action learning sets Study groups Literature search
Shadowing/role models	Critical thinking	Structured evaluative/reflective tool to analyse the situation
Appraisal	Recognition of limitations and areas for development	Production of professional portfolio

The process of assessment as a learning tool ultimately leads to an individual developing the capacity for critical self-evaluation, raising the standards of their own knowledge and skills (Brew, 1999). However, this does not assume that everyone, particularly in the earlier stages of their professional career, has the capacity to do this. It is learnt, modelled by others, and awakened by the power of a transformative learning experience. As such, habitual action, or thoughtful action without reflection, is transformed into critical, reflective self-evaluation (Mezirow and Associates, 1990). However, even when an individual has acquired these skills, they do require to be invigorated by critical self-reflective 'stretching exercises', a concept first coined by Janesick (1998) to refer to exercises undertaken by qualitative researchers to keep their fieldwork skills refined and highly tuned. Some ideas of how to do this are given in Table 7.6.

Following each exercise in Table 7.6, ask the following questions:

- What did I notice about myself as a result of doing this exercise?
- How did I approach the exercise?
- What was difficult about this exercise?
- What did I learn from this?
- What do I need to learn as a consequence of this? (Janesick, 1998).

Table 7.6 Self-reflective stretching exercises.

Performance review
- Seek a 360 degree performance review carefully evaluating how others perceive you and compare and contrast the different interpretations of your clinical care.
- Assume clinical supervision of another – following a model which offers reciprocal appraisal of performance.

Conferences, meetings, reading
- Expose yourself to alternative or divergent perspectives which challenge you to temporarily suspend your own beliefs, and/or reposition yourself in the light of this experience. Articulate the experience to a critical friend.

Teaching
- Demonstrate a clinical skill and then demonstrate a lesser skill in your personal repertoire (non nursing related). Compare and contrast the experience and the evaluations from those you have taught.

Research
- Critically review a piece of research and identify a way to integrate this into your own practice. Explain this process to a novice on the unit.
- Observe the practice on your unit for one hour on three occasions, specifically looking for behaviour or aspects of the environment that you had not noticed before. What have you noticed? What brought this to your attention? How did you describe this? How did you describe the people, the setting, the environment, the mood? If you could undertake an observation study, what would be the research question you would pose as a result of this exercise?
- Interview someone you know well. Ask them to describe a typical day at work. Can you discover something new? What research questions does this illuminate to examine practice in the unit?

Embrace new challenges
- Write for publication; present a paper at conference: write a reflective account of the experience.
- Take a leadership role for an aspect of practice development on the unit.
- Take up a secondment opportunity or participate in an exchange programme.

For each question do not solely consider your scientific knowledge (propositional knowledge), but also examine the art in your nursing (or professional craft knowledge) and finally consider your personal knowledge. The latter two aspects are important, as personal knowledge can be transformed into professional craft knowledge when the practitioner uses themselves as a therapeutic tool; just as propositional knowledge can be transformed by professional craft knowledge (Higgs *et al.*, 2001). Most exercises require you to seek a critical friend to review or feed back your experience. In this way, reflexive thought is transformed into more critical reflective evaluation, especially if the critical friend provides an environment that can expand, distil and uncover some of your taken-for-granted assumptions or deep-rooted beliefs.

One might expect that a senior colleague could cope with any of the critical self-reflective exercises. However, as has been identified, a practitioner whose performance has become less effective, either through lack of motivation, work–life imbalance, or lost vision of nursing, may regress backwards towards levels of performance that might be expected of more junior colleagues. In this situation, they might need to be taken back through the earlier stages of the process to help them recognise areas that need to be developed to progress towards expertise.

Conclusion

A variety of strategies have been examined for enhancing the quality of assessment for students as well as colleagues. The argument has been made that assessment should be seen as a learning or developmental tool. Any assessor should participate in mentorship training, updates or courses to advance their assessment skills. However, the strategies outlined in this chapter might help assessors to consider some of the broader issues related to learning and assessment, and how being an assessor can ultimately serve to confirm one's own core values, standards and beliefs that underpin our own practice.

The next section of the book addresses how these strategies can be applied to the facilitation of practitioners making learning transitions into new roles within the contemporary and future context of critical care provision.

References

Asbridge J (2003) Jonathan Asbridge speech to 2003 RCN Annual Congress http:ww.rcn.org.uk/news/congress2003/display.php?ID=491&Highlight=1 (accessed 15 March 2005).

Barnett R (1997) Beyond competence. In Coffield F and Williamson B (eds). *Repositioning Higher Education*. Buckingham: SRHE and Open University Press.

Brew A (1999) Towards autonomous assessment: using self assessment and peer assessment. In: Brown S and Glasner A (eds). *Assessment Matters in Higher Education: Choosing and Using Diverse Approaches*. Buckingham: SHRE and Open University Press: 159–171.

Brown S (1999) Assessing practice. In: Brown S and Glasner A (eds). *Assessment Matters in Higher Education: Choosing and Using Diverse Approaches*. Buckingham: SHRE and Open University Press: 95–105.

Burkitt I, Husband C, Mackenzie J, Torn A and Crow R (2001) *Nurse Education and Communities of Practice*. Researching Professional Education Series No 18. London: ENB.

Department of Health (1999) *Making a Difference, Strengthening the Nursing, Midwifery and Health Visiting Contribution to Health and Healthcare*. London: DH.

Duffy K (2003) *Failing Students: A Qualitative Study of Factors that Influence the Decisions Regarding the Assessment of Students' Competence to Practice*. Glasgow: Caledonian Nursing and Midwifery Research Centre, Glasgow Caledonian University.

Duke M (1996) Clinical evaluation difficulties experienced by sessional clinical teachers of nursing. A qualitative study. *Journal of Advanced Nursing* **23**: 408–414.

Endacott R, Scholes J, Freeman M and Cooper S (2003) The reality of clinical learning in critical care settings: a practitioner:student gap? *Journal of Clinical Nursing* **12**: 778–785.

Eraut M (1994) *Developing Professional Knowledge and Competence*. London: Falmer Press.

Gerrish K, McManus M and Ashworth P (1997) *Levels of Achievement: A Review of the Assessment of Practice*. Researching Professional Education Series No. 5. London: ENB.

Gutman S, McCredy P and Heisler P (1998) Student level II fieldwork failure: strategies for intervention. *American Journal of Occupational Therapy* **52**: 143–149.

Higgs J, Titchen A and Neville V (2001) Professional practice and knowledge. In: Higgs J and Titchen A (eds). *Practice Knowledge and Expertise in the Health Professions*. Oxford: Butterworth and Heinemann: 3–9.

Hrobsky P and Kersbergen A (2002) Preceptors' perceptions of clinical performance failure. Research brief. *Journal of Nursing Education* **41**(12): 550–553.

Janesick V (1998) *'Stretching' Exercises for Qualitative Researchers*. Thousand Oaks, CA: Sage.

Jeffrey Y (2000) Using competencies to promote a learning environment in intensive care. *Nursing in Critical Care* **5**(4): 194–198.

Jordan S (1999) Self assessment and peer assessment. In: Brown S and Glasner A (eds). *Assessment Matters in Higher Education: Choosing and Using Diverse Approaches*. Buckingham: SHRE and Open University Press: 172–182.

Lankshear A (1990) Failure to fail: the teacher's dilemma. *Nursing Standard* **4**(20): 35–37.

Magnussen L and Amundson M J (2003) Undergraduate nursing student experience. *Nursing and Health Sciences* **5**: 261–267.

Mezirow J and Associates (1990) *Fostering Critical Reflection in Adulthood. A Guide to Transformative and Emancipatory Learning*. San Francisco: Jossey Bass.

Milligan F (1998) Defining and assessing competence: the distraction of outcomes and the importance of the educational process. *Nurse Education Today* **18**(4): 273–280.

Norman I, Watson R, Murrells T, Calman L and Redfern S (2002) The validity and reliability of methods to assess the competence to practice of pre-registration nursing and midwifery students. *International Journal of Nursing Studies* **39**: 133–145.

Northern Ireland Practice and Education Council for Nursing and Midwifery (NIPEC) (2004) Development Framework for Nursing and Midwifery Consultation Document. Belfast: NIPEC (www.nipec.n-i.nhs.uk).

Phillips T, Schostak J and Tyler J (2000) *Practice and Assessment in Nursing and Midwifery: Doing it for Real*. Researching Professional Education Series No. 16. London: ENB.

Rhodes G and Tallantyre F (1999) Assessment of key skills. In: Brown S and Glasner A (eds) *Assessment Matters in Higher Education: Choosing and Using Diverse Approaches*. Buckingham, SHRE and Open University: 106–121.

Rittman M and Osburn J (1995) An interpretive analysis of precepting an unsafe student. *Journal of Nursing Education* **34**(5): 217–221.

Rolfe G (1997) Science, abduction and the fuzzy nurse, an exploration of expertise. *Journal of Advanced Nursing* **25**: 1070–1075.

Rushforth H and Ireland L (1997) Fit for whose purpose? The contextual forces underpinning the provision of nurse education in the UK. *Nurse Education Today* **17**(6): 437–441.

Scholes J (1998) Socialisation: The Gateway to Learning Unpublished MSc Thesis, University of Manchester.

Scholes J and Albarran J (2005) Failing to fail: facing the consequences of inaction. *Nursing in Critical Care* **10**(3): 113–115.

Scholes J and Endacott R (2002) Evaluation of the effectiveness of educational preparation for critical care nursing (ENB, www.nurses-books.co.uk/info.html).

Scholes J. and Smith M (1997) *Starting Afresh: the Impact of the Critical Care Milieu on Newcomers and Novices*. ITU NDU Occasional Paper Series Number 1 (University of Brighton) [ISBN 1 87 196692 2].

Scholes J, Endacott R and Chellel A (1999) *Diversity and Complexity: a Documentary Analysis and Literature Review of Critical Care Nursing*. Researching Professional Education Series No. 13. London: ENB.

Scholes J, Freeman M, Gray M, Wallis B, Robinson D, Matthews Smith G and Miller C (2004) *Evaluation of Nurse Education Partnership*. www.brighton.ac.uk/inam/research/projects/partnerships_report.pdf.

Titchen A and Higgs J (2001) A dynamic framework for the enhancement of health professional practice in an uncertain world: the practice–knowledge interface. In Higgs J and Titchen A (eds). *Practice Knowledge and Expertise in the Health Professions*. Oxford: Butterworth and Heinemann: 215–226.

Turner P (2005) Executive Officer, Council of Heads and Deans. Personal correspondence, 6 May.

United Kingdom Central Council for Nursing, Midwifery and Health Visiting (1999) *Fitness for Practice*. London: UKCC.

Watson H and Harris B (1999) *Supporting Students in Practice Placements in Scotland*. Glasgow: Department of Nursing and Community Health, Glasgow Caledonian University.

Part 3
New ways of working: the contemporary context for developing expertise

Chapter 8
Competence: the building blocks of professional practice

Introduction

In this chapter I shall argue that competencies are a powerful political tool and the *sine qua non* of the modernisation of critical care services. Competencies function as a lever for workforce redesign and ultimately service reorganisation. It is therefore not surprising that much of the agenda for professional practice learning focuses upon the notion of competence acquisition and assessment. This chapter does not explicitly identify the clinical competencies required for critical care practice as this has been discussed at length elsewhere (e.g. Intercollegiate Board for Training in Intensive Care Medicine, 2001; Scholes and Endacott, 2002; Barrett and Bion, 2005). Rather the intention is to offer a philosophical and political analysis of the impact of competencies as a tool to engender change.

Competence is often presented as the minimum standard of performance. However, in this chapter I argue that competence is core to all stages of development and that the competences expected of an expert are broader, more complex and performed 'autonomously' (see Chapter 9). In addition, 'experts' are often expected to pick up additional spheres of practice, especially where these blur traditional role boundaries. Therefore, an 'expert' in one area may be required to adopt new skills or tasks within their job description and have to acquire expertise in the performance of these new roles. Therefore, even 'experts' have components of their job for which they endeavour to achieve competence rather than expertise. The ever-changing dynamics of critical care, set amidst the agenda for service and workforce reconfiguration, mean that practitioners have to constantly evolve and cultivate new spheres of expertise. Competence acquisition is therefore an habitual feature of professional practice at all stages of development, and this process stimulates progression on to the next stage.

Applying core skills and advancing clinical competence in critical care

The priority when inducting a novice to critical care is to ensure an environment of safety for the patient (Jeffrey, 2000). Critical care is a dynamic environment – novices have to know how to monitor a patient closely and respond immediately to altered conditions to prevent further deterioration or to ease the patient into the next stage of recovery. They also have to demonstrate that they understand the assessment findings and can formulate a diagnosis against which to rationalise subsequent caring interventions which are then skilfully applied.[1]

When a nurse demonstrates that she has the necessary knowledge and skills to carry out a given task, she is said to be competent (British Association of Critical Care Nurses (BACCN), 2003). Competency frameworks have been developed in an attempt to capture all the core elements of critical care practice for practitioners at different stages of their critical care career. This is to enable staff to recognise what they need to achieve in their post as well as describing standards against which that individual can be assessed as competent. Such frameworks isolate the subject knowledge which helps to focus the learning that is required in order for the individual to achieve competence (Little, 2000).

The shift towards competency-based assessment has been driven by policy (DH, 2000a, 2001a; National Audit Commission, 2001). The construction of training packages as core skills and competencies, rather than professional qualifications, sits with the agenda of blending roles that cut across professional boundaries, and fits with the skills escalator concept (DH, 2001a). In this way, an individual who is deemed competent to perform a skill can contribute to the effective and efficient delivery of a seamless service (ibid.) and, where this allows for substitution, can create economic benefits (Manley and Garbett, 2000). This fits with the government's modernisation agenda which requires more staff to work differently (DH, 2000b). Staff are enabled to work differently if they are given the necessary training and are then assessed as competent, and this can go some way towards plugging the skills shortage. Therefore, if staff have new skills, they can participate in the reconfiguration of services and re-engineering of new roles to provide patient-centred services (ibid). However, any discussion on competence has to take into account the complex political issues which surround substitution (see Chapter 9). The next section explores the background which sets these arguments in context.

---

[1] A recent study by Bakalis and Watson (2005) concluded that critical care nurses make more diagnoses about the patient's condition and acted in emergency situations more frequently than their colleagues in medical and surgical wards. They also found that critical care nurses are more likely to mentor students than their medical and surgical colleagues. Therefore, students working alongside a critical care nurse are more likely to be exposed to rapid decision making in a situation where a patient is seriously ill and unstable. These data were gathered in the form of a self-report questionnaire to capture 15 different aspects of decision making (Bakalis and Watson, 2005).

Competence

The definition of competence can be problematic (Milligan, 1998). Indeed, there are as many interpretations of the term as authors who write on the subject (Jeffrey, 2000). Competence can refer to the definable aspects of a job, as a stage in a process, or as a dynamic process. Table 8.1 draws out these key distinctions as they are presented in the literature.

The more contemporary interpretation and operationalisation of competency frameworks tend to sit within the first definition of competence in Table 8.1. There, competency refers to the integration of theory and practice to demonstrate aspects of a job that a client or manager may expect from the practitioner (Eraut, 1994), and describes 'the skills and ability to practise safely and effectively without the need for direct supervision' (UKCC, 1999). A competency is therefore a written statement established by expert opinion (Rebekah and Murphy, 1997)

Table 8.1 Different definitions of competence and competencies.

Competence: as definable elements within a role
- Competence: the capabilities and behavioural skills required of a post holder to perform a job.
- Competency: a single knowledge, skill, attitude or value.
- Competencies: stated outcomes of learning to develop a practitioner for enhanced performance in their job.
- Domain: collective term for a group of developmental competencies in a given aspect of performance (NIPEC, 2004).

Competence as a stage in a process
- The ability to operate in the real world whatever the conditions (Benner, 1982).
- One stage in the continuum of skill acquisition from novice to expert (Benner, 1984).
- Incremental development of clinical understanding, technical skill, organisational ability, and ability to anticipate events. The focus shifts from task organisation and completion to focusing on clinical conditions and management of the patient. The competent practitioner has the ability to be more discriminating in evaluation of performance of other members of the team. There is recognition and better understanding of more complex clinical presentations (Benner *et al.*, 1996).

Competence as a dynamic process
- Competence: an expression of work where 'work itself includes the whole complex process through which individuals learn, judge, make decisions and act to manipulate and transform the human purposes, then critically reflect on the results and begin the process of work again' (Phillips *et al.*, 1994: 79). Such an approach has variously been described as 'holistic competence' (Le Var, 1996) and, where it is related to therapeutic caring relationships, as 'higher order competencies' (McAleer and Hamill, 1997: 99).

and can be used to assess performance against selected indicators and identify areas for further development (NIPEC, 2004).

Claims of competence convey what a person can specifically do without implying capability beyond the area specifically outlined in the competence (Eraut, 1994). Such competences are described by the Department of Health (2003a) as outcome-standard-based statements which describe 'what people need to achieve'. These are distinguished from educational competencies which determine 'what people need to possess' (DH, 2003a). However, the level of specificity of a competence can become tighter especially when this relates to a technical task, and more abstract or generic when it refers to 'softer' skills (Eraut, 1994). When this is compared to the competencies written in career progression, one can see that those written for junior or non-professional staff are far more precise and detailed. Competencies for senior staff tend to be written in more conceptual and broad terms, unless that practitioner is taking on a substitution or delegated role, when the phrasing of the competence or competencies reverts to specific and bounded language.

A final layer in the abstract vs specific construction of competence is the number of practitioners to whom that refers. Increasing the range of contexts, particularly where this includes multicultural variables, requires there to be greater abstraction to accommodate local difference. Ironically, the very reason why core competences are promulgated, to benchmark threshold standards, requires the competencies to be written with greater abstraction to allow for local interpretation thus rendering them wide open to difference in application and standards in performance.

Debate about competence-based approaches

The use of competency-based approaches has been driven by policy and is aimed at developing national threshold standards to assure the public (UKCC, 1999; DH, 2000b). However, Cutler (2000) argues that diverse opinion as to what constitutes competence renders such ambitions simplistic and meaningless.

Competences and competencies have the greatest chance of maintaining a consistent standard, when they are:

- locally devised (in response to specific unit practice);
- based on a review of all the evidence from the literature, and preferably 'gold standard' evidence (Greenhalgh, 1997);

and where:

- the educational provision is standardised and a package of learning is repeated to all the participants;
- the competencies are assessed by the same person (or range of people who co-assess the assessors);
- they prescribe performance indicators (clinical performance and underpinning knowledge); and
- they are aimed at a specific cohort of employees (Jeffrey, 2000).

Although such provision might achieve a high level of internal consistency, it may not translate to national threshold standards. Even when attempts are made to apply these standards within a critical care network, high levels of disagreement can lead to detailed negotiation and change. When these extend nationally, consensus can be elusive.

The issues are complex. However, the greatest chance of success for achieving widespread ownership of the competencies (developmental or training frameworks is through consultation, use of expert panels, and/or nominal groups to verify the competencies (NIPEC, 2004; Barrett and Bion, 2005; McLean *et al.*, 2005). Even when such widespread and labour-intensive strategies are fostered, there can still be opposition either because of differing philosophical views about their purpose, or simply resistance to operating within such a high level of prescription or requirement to revise existing frameworks in use (Flanagan *et al.*, 2000). Consequently, attempts at consultation and consensus building to achieve widespread ownership can falter at the point of implementation. Therefore, most competency packages give some leeway for local interpretation, notably by establishing them as minimum standards for achievement against which further competencies can be determined or by offering the potential inclusion of additional levels of performance (Little, 2000).[2]

Where nationally agreed outcomes have been reached, for example the Advanced Trauma Life Support (ATLS) and Advanced Life Support (ALS) training programmes, the level of prescription is tolerated in favour of a higher level of transferable and equivalent skills in the management of advanced life support. How did they do this? First, there is a whole-systems approach to the rollout of the programmes, and, secondly, the programmes have formalised a well rehearsed and recognised procedure for advanced life support.

Such a template is advocated for the introduction of national (and indeed in some cases, international) competencies, founded on the rationale that they provide a minimum standard of quality assurance, something the public has a right to expect (DH, 2001a, 2003a). Advocates argue that they can promote an effective learning environment (Jeffrey, 2000) and can inform curriculum as well as professional development (DH, 2004; NIPEC, 2004; Barrett and Bion, 2005). Further, their use promotes consistency, transferability and staff mobility, especially where there is a single, explicit framework in use (DH, 2004). In addition, it is suggested that competency frameworks provide equality of opportunity for learning and development (DH, 2004).

However, those who argue against the move toward competencies suggest that they inhibit innovation and stifle practice development and the professional artistry of the practitioner (Watson, 2002) because they are rigid, reductionist and oversimplified representations of the occupation (Gonczi, 1994). An

---

[2] When this extends to international competencies (e.g. Competency-based Training in Intensive Care in Europe, CoBaTrICE), the standards for performance have to allow for country-specific regulation and cultural variation.

additional concern is that they assess competence on the day of assessment, but do not assure future competence under different circumstances (Flanagan *et al.*, 2000). Furthermore, unless specifically designed into the framework, competencies do not necessarily identify progression (McLean *et al.*, 2005).

Detailed competencies, designed to assure greater consistency in what is being assessed, cannot reliably ensure that the level of knowledge to be assessed underpins each competence, nor can they necessary marshal how that competence is to be assessed: through direct observation or other assessment media even when expressly stated (McLean *et al.*, 2005). In an attempt to build in greater consistency and reliability, the competencies become lengthy and burdensome (Eraut, 1994). Furthermore, if the competencies have to be revised in light of the introduction of new frameworks or the addition of innovative practice, this becomes a significantly labour- and time-intensive exercise. As a result so much effort and time are dedicated to competency production and maintenance that less time is made available for other educational or developmental activities (Watson, 2002).

Competency frameworks are political. They are powerful organisers to control, frame and steer the workforce. They are a clear risk-management tool that acts to enhance efficiency, effectiveness and productivity because in principle anyone can perform the competency if they have been assessed as competent to do so. In this way they powerfully shift direction and introduce new working agendas and practices across professions, especially, although not exclusively, when considering substitution and delegation.

Two significant competency frameworks have been introduced which exemplify how such influence can affect future directions in practice and their impact on the generation of other national competency frameworks.

The NHS Knowledge and Skills Framework

The NHS KS Framework is a broad, generic framework (DH, 2004) to be used as part of a development review process in conjunction with the implementation of Agenda for Change (DH, 2003b). These competencies are expressly set to deliver the modernisation agenda. The framework addresses six core dimensions: communication; personal and people development; health, safety and security; service improvement; quality; and equality and diversity. A further 24 specific dimensions are identified that do not apply to all jobs in the NHS and they are grouped under the following headings: health and well being; estates and facilities, information and knowledge; and general (ibid.: 6–7). This framework has an explicit human resources and management agenda which forms the basis of career and pay progression, job evaluation and terms and conditions of employment. It is the dominant framework which subsumes others that articulate with it, for example: regulatory requirements or competences, National Occupational Standards, Quality Assurance Agency (QAA) benchmarks, and other nationally developed competences that have been externally quality assured or approved (ibid.: 5). These are necessary adjuncts because the NHS KSF does not describe the exact knowledge and skills that people need to develop (ibid.: 5). There is no leeway for local interpretation (ibid.: 12), because the framework represents a national agreement which has been negotiated between staff and management representatives. However, the NHS KSF does not include doctors, dentists, and some board level and senior managers (DH, 2004).

The NHS KSF framework has strongly framed the Development Framework for Nursing and Midwifery in Northern Ireland (NIPEC[3], 2004). This is a role development framework to support nurses and midwives in developing competence for best performance and is made up of a series of components including: the generic competency profile; portfolio development and utilisation, the learning activities resource, role development guide, career development, and managing poor performance.

Skills for Health Framework

The second influential framework which will become mainstream is the work undertaken by Skills for Health[4]. They have developed a suite of National Workforce Competence Frameworks in the following areas: cancer; children and young people; coronary heart disease; long-term conditions; mental health; older people; and emergency care (Skills for Health, 2004: 24). The Skills for Health framework (based on the model set out in the National Occupational Standards) makes explicit the work activities that need to be carried out to achieve a particular purpose; the quality standards to which these activities need to be performed; and the knowledge and skills people must have in order to carry out the activities. They are explicitly written from the needs of patients and their carers and therefore 'disregard existing professional or service boundaries' (Skills for Health, 2004: 6).

The National Workforce Competence Frameworks have been developed to work in conjunction with the NHS KSF and are designed to support each other. A computerised system to make explicit the links between the two sets of frameworks has been commissioned. Skills for Health claim that their competence frameworks can be used to undertake service reviews, skill-mix review, and in workforce development, role description and redesign, appraisal, development planning, training programmes and qualifications

---

[3] NIPEC was established on 7 October 2004 under the Statutory Rules, The Health and Personal Social Services (2002 Act) (Commencement) Order (Northern Ireland) SR2002 No. 311 (C. 25). In Northern Ireland the NHS is known as the HPSS (NIPEC, 2004: 2, 5).

[4] Skills for Health operates as a strategic body, working in partnership with health sector workforce development organisations. It is supported by the four UK Health Departments, but the Board also has representatives drawn from the voluntary and independent sector, staff side and senior employer members and finally regulatory bodies. It is licensed by the Department for Education and Skills to develop competences. Its remit is to identify sector workforce needs, promote workforce development, and ensure that education and development are driven by the sector's needs (Skills for Health, 2004: 5).

(through National Qualifications Frameworks), and finally as part of the commissioning of education and training (ibid.: 7). Not all the competences are expected of all practitioners, but the frameworks can be used to map the competences of existing staff to deliver the service in the locality, and to identify and develop new roles or extended roles for staff. The competences can be used to determine the type of training and education needs of staff. Examples of new roles developed in the Emergency Care National Workforce Competence Framework include: Emergency Care Practitioner[5], Paramedic Intermediate Care Support Practitioner[6] and Emergency Nurse Practitioner in a Primary Care Suite[7].

The eagerly awaited team competencies for critical care due for completion in January 2005 were strongly influenced by Skills for Health (Manley, 2005). This has resulted in a framework which organises competency units that are outcome oriented, emphasising action rather than knowledge, but which identifies specific units of competencies related to knowledge and skills. These have been written as competencies that are expected to be delivered by the whole service team rather than by one professional group, but allow for individual contribution to be identified. This can illuminate new areas of working and/or new roles that need to be developed to furnish the service niche, but can also identify areas of overlap. The project team commissioned to undertake the Critical Care Team competencies work will seek to influence the work of Skills for Health but ensure that competencies unique to critical care are made explicit as well as those that can be shared within the Emergency, Urgent and Unscheduled Frameworks devised by Skills for Health.

Faculty of Emergency Nursing Framework

The Faculty of Emergency Nursing (FEN) founded by the RCN provides a career framework and competences defined at three levels. FEN's primary aim is to enable professional accreditation of clinical competency set against standards in the following areas (RCN, 2005):

- emergency care of the older person;
- major incident planning;

---

[5] Emergency Care Practitioner: a community role providing a rapid response to non-life-threatening emergency 999 calls, a selected range of GP out of hours calls and other requests from health and social care professionals (Skills for Health, 2004: 17).

[6] Paramedic Intermediate Care Support Practitioner who undertakes the assessment and where possible treatment of older people in their own residence following minor injury. He or she liaises with other health and social care services to continue follow-up services in the patient's own residence (ibid.: 19).

[7] Emergency Nurse Practitioner in a Primary Care Suite: sees, treats and discharges patients autonomously. Deals with minor injuries and illness within parameters of practice and prescribes using patient group directives. The post-holder can refer to other specialities autonomously. Anyone who attends A&E but could have been treated by a GP is referred to the ENP (ibid.: 20).

- pre-hospital care;
- major trauma management;
- emergency care of the adult;
- emergency care of the person with minor injury or illness;
- emergency care of the child and younger person;
- care of the person with psychological needs.

The Faculty of Emergency Nursing reported that 30 members from universities nationwide had mapped their courses to the FEN competences.

FEN is about developing the speciality and uses peer review and a series of competency statements and standards that mark out career progression from Associate to Fellow in the Faculty (Holt, 2005). This is a national initiative and claims to be the first faculty of nursing in the UK and one of the first in the world (Williams, 2005). The extent to which their work is threatened or in competition with the Skills for Health Emergency Care Framework has yet to be understood. However, the Faculty has defended itself from extinction by mapping its competences against the job descriptions in the Agenda for Change bands (Williams, 2005), thus creating a clear articulation with the NHS KSF.

In summary, the NHS KSF sets out competencies to fulfil the modernisation agenda. The Skills for Health suite of competences are expressly generic health care competences and promote the blending of role boundaries and the creation of new services. The instrument by which Agenda for Change is to be implemented in Northern Ireland (the NIPEC version) has managed to retain a focus on the professional development of nurses and midwives. When we recall what NIPEC stands for (Northern Ireland Practice and Education Council for Nurses and Midwives), this makes considerable sense. It is lamentable that no such equivalent framework has been produced by the statutory organisations in the rest of the UK. This leaves the RCN and their Faculty of Emergency Nursing making a distinct contribution. However, this also leaves the RCN Emergency Care Association at risk, because its success relies upon individual nurses subscribing to it and submitting portfolios of their competence to amass sufficient membership to make the Faculty viable. If they find themselves in direct competition with the Emergency Care National Workforce Competence Framework, an explicit tool to be used by workforce planners and Strategic Health Authorities to design the delivery of services, their future will remain uncertain.

Competence deflation and up-skilling

The examination of competence frameworks thus far has demonstrated how the generation of competences to meet patient needs and services can be used to enable anyone to deliver a service if they are subsequently assessed as competent to deliver that practice (within regulatory or statutory requirements).

Unchecked, practice can be reduced to the sum of the parts, and roles can be restructured and redesigned so that they can be delivered by a practitioner in the most cost-effective and potentially time-efficient fashion. In times of staff shortage, widening access into the health care professions and up-skilling unqualified practitioners through competency assessment seem a pragmatic solution to a perennial problem (McLeod, 2001). Such an approach to expanding the workforce to meet the growing demands for health and social care as the population ages is set out in the Government's concept of the 'skills escalator'.

The Department of Health introduced the concept of the skills escalator in 2001. There are two core aims. The first is to attract more staff into the NHS from wider recruitment sources, and the second is about developing staff to respond to changing health care provision (DH, 2001b). The vision of this approach is that individuals can enter the NHS as a 'porter or a cleaner' and can, if they have the 'desire and ability' to progress up the skills escalator, become a 'chief executive or a consultant' with the 'necessary' training (DH, 2001b: 3).

Lifelong learning is the key to making this vision a reality. However, the notion of reducing practice into component parts, which can be delegated to anyone who is deemed competent to perform those skills, does not go without criticism. First, there is the notion of how the sum of the parts does not make up the whole (Cutler, 2000). That is, something of the professional craft knowledge or artistry is lost when elements of care are disaggregated into competences that are delegated down the skills escalator. Secondly, there is a concern that this can lead to fragmentation which can ultimately inhibit the efficiency and effectiveness of the service unless specifically managed, thereby creating more paper-heavy management, training, supervisory and assessment systems (Field, 1993). Thirdly, 'dumbing down' competences into cookbook procedures belies their complexity and the broader theoretical understanding that informs clinical decision making and intervention (Gonczi, 1994). Finally, there is concern about the impact that all this has on the patient's experience of continuity, quality and therapeutic intervention. It would seem that while we have been concerned about qualification inflation we have paid less attention to competence deflation.

The staffing shortage has resulted in pragmatic solutions. Competency-based assessment does theoretically enable people to be trained to do activities that might otherwise have been considered outside their remit. It ensures that a 'competent' individual is at the bedside where perhaps a bed might have been closed because of lack of staff. Such initiatives are introduced under the banner of policy directives which encourage the development of a more flexible workforce and maximise the potential of health care assistants (DH, 2001b). However, flexibility is discussed elsewhere as being achieved by 'professional staff delegating less skilled and non clinical tasks' to support staff (DH, 2000a). The issue clearly is what constitutes a 'less skilled' task, especially when a competency framework alongside an educational package ensures that individuals are 'skilled up' to perform tasks that might formerly have been considered outwith the remit of an un(professionally) trained workforce (here please note the distinction made between professional training and competency-based training).

This has had an impact on critical care nurses. The delegation of nursing tasks to assistants has largely come about because there are not enough registered and specially trained critical care nurses. The chapter now turns to examine the impact of workforce redesign through competence deflation and the impact this has on critical care nursing practice.

The document *'The Nursing Contribution to the Provision of Comprehensive Critical Care for Adults'* (DH, 2001c) has identified four key stages in the clinical career for critical care practitioners. They are: critical care assistants; registered practitioners (including critical care nurses with a specialist qualification); senior registered practitioners (critical care nurses with 4 years' experience who hold senior posts including sister/charge nurse positions, clinical nurse specialists, network leaders, practice educators and some clinical management posts); and finally, consultant practitioners (ibid.: 10). First, the evolving role of critical care assistants is examined to illustrate some of the critical issues relating to delegating competences.

The role of the support worker in critical care

Hind *et al.* (2000) have argued that as nurses have responded to calls to acquire new skills that might previously have been performed by medical staff, some care provided by nurses will need to be delegated to health care assistants (HCAs). Some feared that fundamental care would be delegated to HCAs and this would result in distancing qualified staff from essential care and would fragment the continuity of care and inhibit holistic care provision (Neenan, 1997). Others have gone further to suggest that the dilution of skill mix could ultimately affect the quality of care delivered to the critically ill patient (Bowman *et al.*, 2003) and because of this qualified nurses have resisted HCAs assuming direct patient care (Chang, 1995; Wainwright, 2002).

In response, advanced support worker roles have been introduced which focus on the acquisition of more technical skills, e.g. processing an arterial blood sample, taking blood from an arterial line for analysing arterial blood gases (Sutton *et al.*, 2004); and assisting in intubation and extubation (McLeod, 2001). Indeed, up-skilling of these practitioners, through competency training, the reframing of their title to critical care assistants, and practice that is defined by protocols, has extended their scope of practice into spheres of activity that may formerly have been considered substitution roles undertaken by qualified critical care nurses for doctors, e.g. removal of endotracheal tubes and monitoring of the patient following the procedure (McGloin and Knowles, 2005). The critical care assistants (CCAs) are required to do these activities under the direct supervision of the lead or senior nurse and the CCAs are further charged with the responsibility to report any change to the qualified nurse (BACCN, 2003): echoes from the past of competencies set out to distinguish performance between enrolled and registered nurses[8] (Statutory Instrument, 1983, No. 873; Rule 18: Appendix 1). The fact the CCA programme lasts for 18 months (McGloin and Knowles, 2005) evokes memories of the enrolled nurse 2-year training. However, the use of NVQ level 3 in care and NVQ units from Operating Department Practitioner (ODP) training (McLeod, 2001) suggests more of a shift towards a technical role than to second-level nurse.

The expanding role of an unregulated group of practitioners is hotly debated (Murray, 2001). This has resulted in wide variation in the way in which HCAs are deployed in intensive care settings (Hogan and Playle, 2000). When this is widened out to an examination of the wider critical care community, there would be even greater diversity, especially when considering critical care without walls. The types of distinction between a more 'standard' HCA role and that of an advanced support worker are illustrated in Table 8.2. This has led to a call for the standardisation of competencies, training and support that HCAs receive and the generation of a national database of education and training to provide a basis for regulation of health care assistants (BACCN, 2003).

Advocates of the CCA roles suggest that, with training and consolidation, the CCA can outperform the newly qualified registered nurse in critical care (Warr, 1998; McLeod, 2001). However, an evaluation of the first CCA programme in London reported that five out of the six participants on the programme have subsequently taken up their pre-registration nursing diploma (McGloin and Knowles, 2005). All six CCAs were lost to the unit, leaving the evaluators concerned about the overall cost to the unit in time and financial outlay for development of the programme and assessment of the CCAs (ibid.). Therefore, although a useful recruitment tool, and an excellent demonstration of the way in which widened access into health care and progression up the skills escalator can work, it leaves those who have heavily invested in the development of the CCAs bereft of a valuable resource to staff their unit.

Factors inhibiting delegation to support workers

Patient contact and realising one's therapeutic potential are the things that keep nurses nursing (Scholes, 2003). Therefore, anything which separates the critical care nurse from the patient's bedside fundamentally alters the way in

---

[8] The EN was expected to assist in the assessment, implementation and evaluation of care, supervised by the RGN. The RGN was the practitioner responsible for health promotion; recognition of situations detrimental to health; and the significance of assessment findings as the basis on which care was planned. The RGN had ultimate responsibility for: care planning, implementation, evaluation and overall management of the care group of patients. These directives were used to design curricula for pupil and student nurse training. From 1 September 1992 all ENs could call themselves RN, as the EN roll was disbanded and all practitioners were recorded on a single professional register. However, the level and field of practice for which the individual had been prepared had to be made explicit (UKCC, 1992).

Table 8.2 Illustration of the diverse range of skills and competencies required of support workers in critical care.

HCA roles (Hind et al., 2000)	Advanced Support Worker roles (Sussex Critical Care Network, 2004)	Examples of Critical Care Assistants' skills (McLeod, 2001)
Administrative/clerical tasks	Processing of an arterial blood sample in a blood gas analyser	Undertaking
Restocking equipment	Aseptic technique, simple dressing	Recording patient monitor observations
Supporting staff with patient care	Setting up nasogastric feeding	Recording mechanical ventilation observations
Preparing, dismantling and cleaning equipment	Assisting with clinical procedures, i.e. insertion of arterial lines, CVP lines.	Suctioning cardiovascularly stable, ventilated patients (subsequently removed: McGloin and Knowles, 2005)
Cleaning and preparation of a bedspace	Assisting in securing an ET tube	
Cleaning and stocking the sluice	Eye and mouth care	Neurological observations and assessment in patients without a cerebral insult
	Setting up a humidified oxygen system	Taking blood samples from arterial lines
	Obtaining a specimen, e.g. urine/faeces/CVP line	Removal of arterial lines
	Preparation of transducer lines	
	Optional units	Preparation of NIPPV, CPAP
	Taking of blood from an arterial line for analysing ABGs	Invasive pressure monitoring
	Preparation of major burns dressings	Assisting in:
	Cleaning the bronchoscope	Intubation
	Obtaining and processing a blood gas sample	Extubation
	Setting up of CPAP circuits	Percutaneous tracheostomy insertion
	Taking observations	Changing of tracheostomy tubes
		Insertion of invasive lines
		Removal of invasive lines
		Patient admission
		Patient transfer (under supervision)

Abbreviations: ABGs, arterial blood gases; CPAP, continuous positive airway pressure; CVP, central venous pressure; ET, endotracheal tube; NIPPV, non-invasive positive pressure ventilation.

which the nurse formulates clinical judgements about that patient and subsequently interacts with them. This may account for resistance among qualified nurses to CCAs doing measuring and recording of observations and fluid balance (Ramprogus and O'Brien, 2002; Gray, 2003). The issue is in the way in which nurses consistently read physiological data and change parameters to progress the patient. Reading, thinking, formulating judgements and acting happen in an iterative and sometimes seamless fashion. Delegating this activity to an assistant serves only to disrupt this process. Rather than being resource efficient, it serves to be resource intensive, not only in the requirement to train and up-skill the assistants in the first place, but also because, when assistants are required to defer all decisions to the qualified nurse, this can result in duplication of effort. The following examples illustrate this potential problem.

The transition from professor to HCA

In the Autumn of 2004 I was given the exceptional privilege of being allowed to return to intensive care and undertake 12 days of supervised clinical practice. It had been decided, in negotiation with the clinical manager of the department, that within the restricted time frame, and given the fact that it was 25 years since I had practised in critical care, we should realistically set my learning outcomes. Recently, the department had introduced a set of advanced HCA competencies in negotiation with the local critical care network (Sutton *et al.*, 2004). It was decided that I should seek to achieve these. Normally an HCA would be given a period of six months to do this, with flexibility to take longer if required, because the premise was that the postholder should only be assessed when they felt confident in their knowledge and skills. However, I was given 'advanced standing' for my past clinical work as well as recent time spent observing practice in ITU as a researcher, and the time frame was collapsed down to 12 days.

I felt it was critical for me to get back into practice and see if I could still do what I write about and advocate. It felt very important to experience the real world of clinical delivery as a complete participant, rather than in my more familiar recent role as observer-as-participant (Gold, 1958). I realise this was extremely time limited and very tightly supervised. I also probably had far greater power and control over the situation by dint of my position in the local HEI but at no stage did I need to flex my academic muscle to demand a greater level of supervision. Although some senior staff with whom I had worked as a teacher or researcher showed some reservations about my shift to HCA in practice, the HCAs and receptionists did not hold back in their criticism that I was 'only playing at it'. However, I genuinely intended to fully engage in practice and felt quite wounded by their painful assault on the truth: indeed in 12 days how could I achieve anything more than 'playing at it'? I wrote a reflective diary during this time and some of these observations have been used here to examine some of the potential dynamics that might exist between HCAs and qualified staff. The first scenario shows how an

HCA doing fundamental care might impede clinical decision making; and the second illustrates how delegating the task of recording observations to an advanced critical care support worker might be resisted by qualified staff.

Scenario 8.1:   Reflecting on delegating fundamental care

It was quaintly observed how meticulous I was in attending to mouth care[9]. I have long considered the things that nurses do often relate to their own particular 'pet hates'. Mine are dry cracked lips and cold feet. Hence if I found my patient had cold feet (after ensuring this was not due to circulatory collapse) I would wrap them in orthopaedic padding, leaving one toe visible to assess changes in colour. I cleaned mouths on a regular basis and routinely applied Vaseline to the patient's lips to keep them moist. This is not to suggest I neglected the toothbrush. I judiciously applied toothpaste to brush and cleaned round the mouth, scraped the tongue and then moistened off afterwards with swabs, finally carefully suctioning any additional fluid caught at the back of the mouth. However, I freely admit I reached for the mouth care tray every time I got scared. Fortunately a patient was never placed at risk when this happened as there was always a staff nurse supervising me who could take over the technical side. On reflection, I recognise this was 'old school' interventionism! I acted with similar fastidiousness when it came to eye care because some things are so deeply rooted.

When I stepped back into practice, I had to own up to the fact that my perspective on what constituted high quality care in critical care was about a sound technical knowledge base, applied through attentive presence and hypervigilance of change. By attending to fundamental care, I felt able to use these encounters with the patient to reassess, make decisions, and assure the patient of my presence. Fundamentally, these values had grown from my past experience as a critical care nurse, but had been refined through my teaching and research. But I was locked in the time warp of the high standards of care that had been taught to me and the effects of exposure to practice assessments and evaluations of my past performance by colleagues and most importantly patients and their relatives. The point was that, to effectively enable my transition to contemporary practitioner, these values would need to be blended with current exemplars of excellence in critical care nursing (and of course my personal assessment of when they occurred naturally went through my perceptual filter). To do that I would need time to rehearse and consolidate new skills and learn an adapted way of working under the close supervision of a

---

[9] I recognised that I was resorting to clinical performance which made me feel safe as much as I hoped it was providing comfort to the patients. The important issue is to enable practitioners to be able to achieve technical competence at the same time as maintaining core values and standards in fundamental care practice. The two are not mutually exclusive.

well practised critical care nurse. However, there was a danger that my interventions were seen to be an implicit criticism of my colleagues' standards of care. I return to an excerpt from my reflective diary to further examine this.

Scenario 8.2: Reflecting on implicit criticism?

Although my academic role had been temporarily suspended, some supervisors were concerned that my actions (attending to fundamental care and being consciously present at the side of the patient) were an implicit criticism of their standards of care. Indeed, many asked me to step back and review the computer screen (patient data) and care plans, to emphasise (or, it seemed, to assure me) that they had dealt with all the patient's priorities. I was attending to the fundamental care because I felt this was the way I could make a contribution as it enabled them to be free to attend to the patient's other needs. My supervisors commented that my actions demonstrated initiative and this distinguished me from other students who might be far more passive. Further, they stated that they found me to be 'very caring' and this served to remind them that perhaps they should consciously attend to these aspects of care with greater regularity. However, I quickly learnt to make explicit the motivation for my actions and asked them to specify when they required me to do something else to assist them. I also quickly learnt to reflexively re-position myself if I sensed some irritation. This had been learnt from the experience of being a fieldworker, notably through the role of observer-as-participant, which made me highly tuned in to signs that I was causing a disturbance to their practice.

By dint of my position, greater tolerance was afforded me. My behaviour was reviewed by some with suspicion: why would someone seek to make the transition from a position of privilege to one of subservience? Was I, in fact, under cover? When assured that I had no such intention, I was passed off as an eccentric. I was tolerated because my presence was temporary and supernumerary, and they did not have to invest in the development of a future member of staff. But this left me to wonder how this might impact upon the relationship between a qualified nurse and an HCA, if the HCA role had been designed expressly to do these tasks on behalf of the qualified nurse on a daily basis.

Scenario 8.3: Delegating observational tasks to the HCAs

The next phenomenon of distinction was the presence of computers by the bedside. These constantly recorded patient data. Each hour the nurse had to verify the data and cross-reference/check against the data displayed on the monitor. Unfortunately, the computers were situated to one side of the bed space. This had been done to wire the computers into the local network, and reduce hazards of tripping over associated leads. However, this served to locate the workstation in a position that invariably required the nurse to turn their back to the patient. It was also placed at a distance that meant the nurse could not maintain contact with the patient when working on the computer. Recent stringent infection control policy identified the keyboard as a potential source of cross-infection, and therefore physical contact with the patient had to be concluded (with gloves removed and hands washed) before touching the keyboard. This seemed to reduce the amount of time the nurses spent in direct physical contact with their patients.

This to me was a sad indictment of the times. Previous research (Scholes and Moore, 1997) had illuminated the therapeutic impact of contact with the patient and demonstrated that some expert nurses were able to reach a deeply agitated patient and bring calmness and alleviate their distress by the use of touch and by assuring the patient of their presence. I saw less of this on my recent return to practice. This was not to say it was absent: it was more to do with seeing fewer staff doing this on a regular basis. There are a number of factors that could have caused this, not least of which was the original observation about how much sicker the patients seemed to be (which I would have hoped would have increased the incidence of therapeutic presence rather than diminishing it). Secondly, I noticed a predisposition among staff to change the ventilatory settings and titrate medication and fluids, leaving little time for the patient to 'settle' with a nurse in contact with the patient and for vigilantly observing changes to the patient's parameters. A conversation with a sage intensive care sister with many decades of experience on the notion of 'watchful waiting' indicated that this area of expertise was on the decline. Increasingly, staff were encouraged to progress the patient, sometimes quite aggressively, in line with the weaning protocol. This meant that staff were also quick to change settings to increase support if the patient did not seem to respond immediately. This seemed to result in considerable 'bounce' in the patient's response.

In another conversation with a neighbour who recently returned to ITU practice after seven years, we mused on the notion of whether we considered this to be *too much* 'fiddling'. We were quite quizzical about this on the basis of our 'outdated' potentially 'old school' perspectives, especially when we were assured that this behaviour was about progressing the patient through their care pathway.

This vignette serves to illustrate how important it is for qualified staff to undertake the observations and maintain control of the patient's fluid balance, and why there might be a great reluctance to delegate these tasks to the HCA or CCA (Wainwright, 2002). Essentially, staff were responding immediately to changed parameters in the patient's observations, either to progress the patient or to increase support if there wasn't a suitable response. The introduction of a third party to record the findings and then report these to a qualified nurse, who would then guide the CCA on what to do, would actually impede a fluid, iterative process of assessment, intervention and evaluation. Furthermore, if an HCA constantly approached a qualified nurse who was caring for her own patient, it would only serve to distract her conscious attention on her own assessment–intervention–evaluation cycle. Furthermore, an HCA/CCA would not be able to make changes to the patient's ventilatory settings or fluids, requiring the qualified nurse to attend the second patient and undertake her own assessment–intervention–evaluation cycle. Thereby, the work would be duplicated rather than delegated.

The notion of watchful waiting as an exemplar of expertise relates back to Benner's description of the expert practitioner who, with a repertoire of experience, has a 'clinical grasp' of the situation that enables them to iden-tify illness trajectories (Benner *et al.*, 1996: 147). This influences the expert's response, because they can read when to 'jump in' and when to 'hold back' (ibid.: 158). Their experience allows them to zero in on a problem, recognising altered cues to effect an immediate response that is uncluttered by alternative diagnoses and solutions (Benner, 1984). However, close intervention with the patient, and understanding their specific response to situations and interven-tions, help to refine their ability to do this. Delegating this to others makes the knowledge of that person second hand. Benner *et al.* (1996) suggest that the expert nurse has 'expanded peripheral vision', which can take into account the needs of patients on the units and recognise where other nurses might be struggling (ibid.: 154). This would suggest that any CCA who had a patient allocated to them would require the supervision of an expert to maximise the potential of their contribution. Every unit has an expert – some may be lucky to have several – but it is doubtful as to whether or not less experienced staff could easily incorporate the supervision of CCA practice within their daily practice.

These role are new. Rigorous evaluation of their impact needs to be under-taken that takes into account the experience for practitioners in the CCA role and those who supervise them, as well as the patient experience. Also, the range of competencies and the level of education and support that are required to meet the requisite knowledge and skills call for careful monitoring.

Conclusion

Competency frameworks and the assessment of competence have been used to re-engineer services and enable new workers to work differently. Compet-ences are important frameworks to assure the public that practitioners have the requisite set of skills to enable them to perform at a minimum standard of safety. In highly technical environments they are invaluable to help induct staff in the use of new devices, protocols or procedures. However, they can be extremely limiting or so costly in time and effort to update that they become burdensome and this limits attention to other possible areas of practice development.

Competency frameworks have been used to define the expected clinical competency of a range of health care workers (McLeod, 2001). However, they have been instrumental in the delegation of tasks or blurring of role boundaries. Rarely if ever does one see the updraft of a competence to a senior colleague in another health care profession (although physicians' protests to restore certain competencies to be within the sole province of a medical practitioner are frequently heard). Therefore, competence assessment tends to be specifically designed to facilitate the substitution of roles as much as to assure the public of a basic standard of care as a consequence of a qualification. Poor standards of care have contributed to the managerial response to produce more competencies. The crisis in confidence about the failure of educational provision to provide practitioners who were fit for purpose has also resulted in the commissioning and design of educational programmes reshaped around competencies.

In clinical practice, time constraints and an inadequate staffing resource have all contributed to the demand for the delegation of competences. Education has been charged with the responsibility to set up training programmes to prepare practitioners to meet these new roles. Often these programmes have been designed at considerable speed. The only thing faster is the time frame in which the individual is expected to undertake the necessary learning to fit them for their new role. To add to this complexity, it is often a challenge to find a sufficient number of suitably qualified practitioners to supervise and undertake the number of assessments required to confer competence on the individual practitioner, especially where there is large demand, e.g. comprehensive physical assessment modules which are subject to excessive oversubscription by practitioners who are taking up community matron roles or contributing to Hospital at Night services.

Importantly, as competences are delegated to senior nurses, they too have to delegate part of their role to support workers. This leads to a constant reshuffle of who does what and when, otherwise known as modernising. This can obscure the reason why a practitioner might consider an intervention core to their role and why delegation might create duplication in effort. It is therefore essential that critical care nurses clearly articulate the essence of their practice that makes up the whole of what they do, and not focus solely upon the more easily definable constituent parts that make up a series of competencies. That is why, throughout this book, strategies to facilitate the articulation of the essence of nursing and how to enable practitioners to realise their full therapeutic potential have been addressed. Strategies to achieve transformational learning and therapeutic care must be in place to help scaffold the essential functional competence-based component of any critical care role. The critically ill patient deserves no less from the practitioners who provide their treatment and care.

The modernising project is dependent on the delegation of competences but can only be considered a success if this does not increase risk and receives positive patient evaluation. Therefore, we must be sure that research and evaluation of all these new roles are robust and include listening to the voices of patients and their relatives.

In the next chapter John Albarran explores the impact of competence delegation from traditional medical roles into 'advanced nursing roles', and compares these substitution roles with ones that embrace new competencies to enhance autonomous nursing practice and patient services.

References

Bakalis N and Watson R (2005) Nurses' decision-making in clinical practice. *Nursing Standard* **19**(23): 33–39.

Barrett H and Bion J (2005) An international survey of training in adult intensive care medicine. *Intensive Care Medicine* **31**: 553–561.

Benner P (1982) Issues in competency-based testing. *Nursing Outlook* **30**: 303–309.

Benner P (1984) *From Novice to Expert*. California, Addison-Wesley.

Benner P, Tanner C and Chesla C (1996) *Expertise in Nursing Practice: Caring, Clinical Judgement and Ethics*. New York: Springer.

Bowman S, Bray K, Leaver G, Pilcher T, Plowright C and Stewart L (2003) Health care assistants' role, function and development: results of a national survey. *Nursing in Critical Care* **8**: 141–148.

British Association of Critical Care Nurses (BACCN, 2003) Position statement on the role of health care assistants who are involved in direct patient care activities within critical care areas. *Nursing in Critical Care* **8**: 3–12.

Chang A (1995) Perceived functions and usefulness of health support workers. *Journal of Advanced Nursing* **21**: 67–74.

Cutler L (2000) Competence in context. *Nursing in Critical Care* **5**: 294–299.

Department of Health (2000a) *The NHS Plan: a Plan for Investment, a Plan for Reform* (available at: http://www.doh.gov.uk/nhsplan/nhsplan.htm).

Department of Health (2000b) *Comprehensive Critical Care: A Review of Adult Critical Care Services*. London: DH.

Department of Health (2001a) *Working Together – Learning Together – A Framework for Lifelong Learning for the NHS*. London, DH.

Department of Health (2001b) The Skills Escalator Information Pack (available at http://www.doh.gov.uk/hrinthenhs/learning/).

Department of Health (2001c) *The Nursing Contribution to the Provision of Comprehensive Critical Care for Adults: A Strategic Programme of Action*. London: HMSO.

Department of Health (2003a) *The NHS Knowledge and Skills Framework (NHS KSF) and Development Review Guidance* – working draft. London: DH.

Department of Health (2003b) *Agenda for Change – Proposed Agreement*. London: HMSO.

Department of Health (2004) *The NHS Knowledge and Skills Framework (NHS KSF) and Development Review Process*. London: HMSO.

Eraut M (1994) *Developing Professional Knowledge and Competence*. London: Falmer Press.

Field J (1993) Competency and the pedagogy of labour. In Thorpe M, Edwards R and Hanson A (eds). *Culture and Processes of Adult Learning*. London: Routledge: 39–50.

Flanagan J, Baldwin S and Clarke D (2000) Work-based learning as a means of developing and assessing nursing competence. *Journal of Clinical Nursing* **9**: 360–368.

Gold R (1958) Field relations. In McCall G and Simmons J (eds). *Issues in Participant Observation: a Textbook and Reader*. Boston, MA: Addison Wesley.

Gonczi A (1994) Competence based assessment in the professions in Australia. *Assessment in Education* **1**(1): 27–44.

Gray J (2003) Why nurses may be reluctant to step aside. *Nursing Standard* **18**: 3.

Greenhalgh T (1997) *How to Read a Paper: the Basics of Evidence-based Medicine*. London: BMJ Publishing Group.

Hind M, Jackson D, Andrews C, Fulbrook P, Galvin K and Frost S (2000) Health care support workers in the critical care setting. *Nursing in Critical Care* **5**: 31–39.

Hogan J and Playle J (2000) The utilisation of the healthcare assistant role in intensive care. *British Journal of Nursing* **8**: 794–801.

Holt L (2005) Emergency Care Association Position Statement on the Faculty of Emergency Nursing. http://www.rcn.org.uk/faculty (accessed 16 April 2005).

Intercollegiate Board for Training in Intensive Care Medicine (ICBTICM, 2001) The CCST in Intensive Care Medicine: Competency-based Training and Assessment. www.qmc.nhs.uk/aicu/Documents/part1.doc (accessed 17 April 2005).

Jeffrey Y (2000) Using competencies to promote a learning environment in intensive care. *Nursing in Critical Care* **5**(4): 194–196.

Le Var R (1996) NVQs in nursing, midwifery and health visiting: a question of assessment and learning? *Nurse Education Today* **16**: 85–93.

Little C (2000) Technological competence as a fundamental structure of learning in critical care nursing: a phenomenological study. *Journal of Clinical Nursing* **9**: 391–399.

Manley K (2005) Changing context impacts competencies project. *Critical Care Mail*. RCN Critical Care Forum, winter 2004/2005: 7.

Manley K and Garbett R (2000) Paying Peter and Paul: reconciling concepts of expertise with competency for a clinical career structure. *Journal of Clinical Nursing* **9**: 347–359.

McAleer J and Hamill C (1997) *The Assessment of Higher Order Competence Development in Nurse Education*. County Antrim: University of Ulster.

McGloin S and Knowles J (2005) An evaluation of the critical care assistant role within an acute NHS Trust critical care unit. *Nursing in Critical Care* **10**(4): 210–215.

McLean C, Monger E and Lally I (2005) Assessment of practice using the NHS Knowledge and Skills Framework. *Nursing in Critical Care* **10**(3): 136–142.

McLeod A (2001) Critical care assistants: from concept to reality. *Nursing in Critical Care* **6**(4): 175–181.

Milligan F (1998) Defining and assessing competence: the distraction of outcomes and the importance of educational process. *Nurse Education Today* **18**: 273–280.

Murray K (2001) Invaluable assistance. *Nursing Standard* **16**: 12.

National Audit Commission (2001) *Hidden Talents: Education, Training and Development of Healthcare Staff in the NHS Trusts*. London: Audit Commission.

Neenan T (1997) Advanced practitioners: the hidden agenda? *Intensive and Critical Care Nursing* **13**: 80–86.

Northern Ireland Practice and Education Council for Nursing and Midwifery (NIPEC, 2004) *Development Framework for Nursing and Midwifery*. Consultation Document. Belfast: NIPEC (www.nipec.n-i.nhs.uk).

Phillips T, Bedford H, Robinson J and Schostack L (1994) *Education, Dialogue and Assessment: Creating Partnerships for Improved Practice*. London: ENB.

Ramprogus V and O'Brien D (2002) The case for formal education of HCAs. *Nursing Times* **28**: 37–38.

Rebekah N and Murphy J (1997) Legal and practical impact of clinical practice guidelines on nursing and medical practice. *The Nurse Practitioner* **22**: 138–148.

Royal College of Nursing (2005) The Faculty of Emergency Nursing. www.rcn.org.uk/faculty (accessed 16 April 2005).

Scholes J (2003) The Skills Escalator: implications for critical care nursing. *Nursing in Critical Care* **8**(3): 93–95.

Scholes J and Endacott R (2002) *Evaluation of the Effectiveness of Educational Preparation for Critical Care Nursing.* ENB via NMC website www.nmc-uk.org [ISBN 1 901 697 770].

Scholes J and Moore M (1997) *Making a Difference: the Way in which the Nurse Interacts with the Critical Care Environment and Uses Herself as a Therapeutic Tool.* ITU NDU Occasional Paper Series No. 2 (University of Brighton) [ISBN 1 87196679 5].

Skills for Health (2004) *Emergency Care National Workforce Competence Framework Guide.* Bristol: Skills for Health.

Sussex Critical Care Network (2004) *Critical Care Nursing Assistant Competencies.* Unpublished assessment document, Brighton Adult Intensive Care Unit.

Sutton J, Valentine J and Rayment K (2004) Staff views on the extended role of health care assistants in the critical care unit. *Intensive and Critical Care Nursing* **20**: 249–256.

United Kingdom Central Council for Nursing, Midwifery and Health Visiting (1992) The new title 'Registered Nurse'. *Register* **11**: 6.

United Kingdom Central Council for Nursing, Midwifery and Health Visiting (1999) *Fitness for Practice.* London: UKCC.

Wainwright T (2002) The perceived function of health care assistants in intensive care: nurses' views. *Intensive and Critical Care Nursing* **18**: 171–180.

Warr J (1998) An evaluative study into the effectiveness of level 3 national vocational qualification support staff to nurses. *Nurse Education Today* **18**: 505–516.

Watson R (2002) Clinical competence: Starship Enterprise or straitjacket? *Nurse Education Today* **22**: 476–480.

Williams G (2005) 2005 is filled with exciting opportunity. *Emergency Care Association Newsletter* spring: 2.

Chapter 9
New roles in critical care practice

John W. Albarran

Introduction

This chapter examines the extension, expansion and development of new roles within critical care nursing as a response to changing provision. The emergence of new roles in health care and nursing is complex and cannot be attributed to one single factor. The interaction between National Health Service policies, government initiatives, health care technology, professional drivers and demographic trends has collectively challenged traditional models of patient management and care delivery (see Chapter 3). Effective health care includes exploring and improving the delivery of services through new treatments and interventions in novel settings. This entails new ways of working, new roles and reviewing workforce knowledge and skills.

This chapter also critically examines the nature and consequence of these emerging roles for critical care nursing. A central focus of discussion is whether such roles genuinely augment nursing's contribution to patient care or whether they are merely doctor substitution. In addition, the chapter considers the implications for patient care and asks whether all existing roles may be described as advanced practice by evaluating current concepts and criteria developed by national and international bodies.

New roles: the early background

Reviewing governmental policy from the 1970s indicates a strong commitment to expanding the skills of nurses. This period of nursing witnessed many practice and education developments which raised awareness that, to fulfil certain clinical posts, nurses needed a wider knowledge and skills base (Albarran and Fulbrook, 1998). The expansion of specialist hospitals (e.g. oncology and mental health care) increased this demand further. As these roles became more established, the Royal College of Nursing (RCN, 1988) championed the formal recognition of specialist nurses provided that individuals met a set of specified criteria that included practice, education and research. The United Kingdom Central Council's (UKCC, 1990) Post-Registration Education and Preparation for Practice Project (PREPP) subsequently introduced three levels of practice: primary, advanced and consultant, to distinguish between the knowledge and skills that nurses gained and developed through education and clinical experience. At the advanced and consultant level, it was expected that these nurses would be able to exercise clinical discretion and accept greater responsibility. Benner's (1984) work illustrated that nurses' practice progressed from a novice stage to an expert level by developing a repository of clinical skills and expertise. This expertise allows for differentiation between individual nurses regarding their ability to recognise subtle changes in patients' well-being, and to problem-solve and make decisions. This was reinforced by the introduction of the *Scope of Professional Practice* (SoPP) (UKCC, 1992a). SoPP established a framework that enabled nurses, midwives and health visitors to extend and develop their skills provided this was in the interests of patient care. This combination of drivers engineered a model of practice which strengthened all levels of autonomy and accountability and paved the way for nurses to meet people's health care needs in new and imaginative ways (Albarran and Fulbrook, 1998).

The context of new roles – extension, expansion and development

The development of new roles in health care has been complex. Cameron (2000) has identified three key factors, but there are other aspects that cannot be neglected in this discourse:

- the impact of health service reforms;
- the impact of government initiatives;
- changes in the delivery of health services;
- professional expectations;
- blurring and blending policies.

The impact of health service reforms

Specific legislation arising from NHS reforms has influenced the emergence of new roles in nursing (Read, 1998; Cameron, 2000). For example, The NHS and Community Care Act (1990) transferred budgetary powers to each NHS Trust, enabling financial affairs to be managed locally. To control budgets, many Trusts scaled down the size of their workforce by grade-mix reviews, introduced competitive tendering for domestic services and created new professional roles, for example nurse-led anaesthetic clinics, patient discharge and follow-up clinics. These were aimed at improving services and reducing costs.

The ability of NHS Trusts to determine their skill-mix, and the introduction of SoPP (1992), have been regarded as influential forces in the development of new roles in nursing (Read, 1998). General practitioners were also given powers to develop primary care and purchase services from acute NHS Trusts. They were now able to demand that specialist services be delivered in GP surgeries rather than in hospitals and to introduce additional health services for their patients. Through such mechanisms, GPs were able to influence the work of other practitioners and determine the evolution of certain roles such as asthma and diabetic nurses. *The New NHS: Modern, Dependable* (DH, 1997) revised the way primary care services were commissioned, and nurses were seen as having key management and leadership roles because of their position and understanding of community priorities (Cameron, 2000).

More recently, the National Service Framework (NSF) for Coronary Heart Disease (DH, 2000a) was introduced to modernise cardiac services by improving accessibility and delivery of cardiac services. Areas for change included reducing cigarette smoking, improving the management and treatment of patients with coronary heart disease and increasing rehabilitation services. Nurses are one group of health care workers who have responded positively to these challenges. For example, in those suspected of an acute myocardial infarction (AMI), the recommendations stated that thrombolysis should be administered within 20 minutes following admission to hospital (DH, 2000b). The time between arrival in hospital to the administration of thrombolysis is critical to outcomes of survival and is used as a benchmark for assessing performance. To meet the proposed 'door-to-needle times', initiatives such as nurse-practitioner led thrombolysis, acute chest pain nurse, and nurse-led and initiated thrombolysis have been introduced (Albarran, 2004). The impact of these posts has translated to improved patient outcomes. The NSF also recommended that NHS Hospital Trusts introduce protocols and procedures to improve the management and delivery of cardiac services including the wide-scale introduction of chest pain clinics (DH, 2000b). The launch of the NSF chapter on 'Arrhythmias and sudden death' (DH, 2005) is likely to generate dedicated roles to support and educate patients and families about conditions and treatments (Martins *et al.*, 2004). Overall, successive NHS reforms and government policies have encouraged the implementation of new roles and challenged nursing to identify innovative ways of delivering patient care effectively and efficiently (DH 1997, 1998, 1999a, 2000b).

The impact of government initiatives

A key development promoting new roles and ways of working within health care was *The New Deal* (NHS Management Executive, 1991; Read *et al.*, 1999; Rushforth and Glasper, 1999). This directive reduced the number of hours worked by junior doctors which, coupled with shortages in specialities such as anaesthetics, created gaps in service provision that could be addressed by nurses (Read, 1998). Trusts responded by employing nurses and other health care professionals (HCPs) in creative ways to meet the staff shortages. Funding was also made available to support developments. Many NHS Trusts used this to implement nurse-led pre-operative surgical clinics and medical admission nurse specialists (Murray *et al.*, 1995; Doyal *et al.*, 1998) to fill the gaps left as a result of *The New Deal* (NHS Management Executive, 1991). While some of these posts enhanced continuity of care and eased the workload of medical staff, the effect on patient outcomes was never evaluated (Cameron, 2000). Over the years there has been growing resentment amongst nurses that has emerged from an unchallenged assumption that they would unconditionally assume tasks that doctors wished to discard from their practice (Rushforth and Glasper, 1999). Changes in junior doctors' hours are still viewed by half of NHS hospital nurses as responsible for workload increases (Ball and Pike, 2005). Likewise changes in GP contracts have led to a rise in the amount of out-of-hours care provided by community nurses.

The evolution of nursing roles was also influenced by other mandates such as the introduction of waiting list initiatives which followed intense public criticisms (Cameron, 2000). To ameliorate the situation, the Government issued guidance that no patients should wait more than two years on a hospital waiting list (DH, 2000b). One hundred medical consultants were appointed and £33 million was available to cover this. NHS Trusts were expected to implement their strategies to reduce waiting lists or suffer financial penalties. Many Trusts increased patient throughput by running routine surgery at weekends. Other innovations included the appointment of nurses and other HCPs to specific roles so that surgeons could spend more time in the operating theatre. For example, nurses were trained as surgeon's assistants to perform specific surgical procedures and investigations (Royal College of Surgeons in England, 1999; Boss, 2002). Typically, these new roles involved therapeutic or diagnostic duties previously outside the remit of nursing (Bowey and Caballero, 1996). Role transition has not been smooth, for example nurses working in walk-in centres undertake many functions previously performed by GPs yet many feel inadequately prepared (Rosen and Mountford, 2002).

Turning to critical care, *Comprehensive Critical Care* (DH, 2000c) proposed a radical service restructuring and modernisation of health care provision by dismantling the existing boundaries between professional groups and specialities to focus on patient needs. This was precipitated by a series of 'winter crises' in which critically ill patients were transferred to other hospitals due to a lack of intensive care unit (ICU) beds within their locality. To avoid relocating patients, some units discharged highly dependent cases to inadequately prepared wards. The national capacity of ICU and high dependency units was felt to be inadequate. In support of these claims, a series of studies concluded that care on wards was suboptimal and that many deaths could be avoided by additional training and skill development (Morgan *et al.*, 1997; Garrard and Young, 1998; Goldhill *et al.*, 1998). Some ICU nurses, in new roles, were beginning to address these areas (Coad and Haines, 1999).

Funding to the value of £142 million was provided as part of the modernisation programme (Cuthbertson, 2003). Apart from increasing the number of beds, the funds were also to support proposals within *Comprehensive Critical Care* (DH, 2000c) such as introducing multidisciplinary critical care outreach teams to raise the standard of care received by critically ill ward patients. These teams were formed of highly skilled practitioners and were responsible for averting intensive care unit admissions, for following up patients from ICU/HDU and sharing skills with ward staff (Coombs and Dillon, 2002).

Like other reforms, comprehensive critical care reshaped the landscape of intensive care practice and precipitated the growth of new roles. One problem of outreach teams is that experienced staff have been recruited to join (Coombs and Dillon, 2002) or to establish new educational roles (Murch and Warren, 2001). This has left many ICUs short of experienced staff.

The needs for cost containment are inextricably linked with NHS priorities for maximising patient throughput and reducing waiting lists. Other similar schemes, such as heart failure and CHD clinics, have employed nurses to provide health education and information about medication, self-monitoring, and risk factor modification (West *et al.*, 1997; Cline *et al.*, 1998; Blue *et al.*, 2001; Strömberg, 2002; Raftery *et al.*, 2005). However, the focus of new roles has been questioned. Concern over the direction and medical emphasis of many roles have led Brown (1995) and Salussolia (1997) to warn nurses to exercise caution when implementing new roles that do not encompass a holistic framework of care. It could be argued that, if nurses had played a decisive part in the design of new roles, they might have been planned systematically to include a nursing perspective with integrated assessment of competence (Cameron, 2000). The lack of coherence can be seen in the diversity of posts described in the literature (Scholes *et al.*, 1999; Roberts-Davis and Read, 2001). Typically roles were implemented in the absence of a clear definition of boundaries, career pathways and professional development (Levenson and Vaughan, 1999). This has affected transitional arrangements for new post-holders, and many nurses feel insecure about their ability to succeed (Briggs, 1997; Gibson and Bamford, 2001; Lloyd Jones, 2005).

The vignettes below are based on real situations but have been altered to maintain confidentiality. They exemplify a legacy of disorganisation in which post-holders were appointed into advanced/practitioner roles without any form of approved preparation. These nurses' careers and their completion of short courses have favoured competency training to meet service needs. Nursing has inherited a large number of titles without clear roles, boundaries and scope for practice, adding to the confusion over practice roles (Thompson and Watson, 2005).

Scenario 9.1

I am currently a nurse practitioner working in nephrology. My previous post was as a senior sister in nephrology which I did for three years in a regional centre. I do not have a degree, but I completed a Research in Practice course run by the RCN at level 2 in 1999. Prior to this I completed the ENB 136 in renal nursing and have 8 years' experience in this field. In addition I have undertaken a diploma in counselling but this is not university accredited.

As a nurse practitioner, my role is autonomous and currently I am learning how to administer drugs, with the view to having my own CAPD clinic and supporting patients awaiting kidney transplants. I am also currently managing patients in the community who are receiving dialytic therapies for their chronic renal conditions. A substantial amount of my time is teaching and development, I have taught at the local university on diploma and degree programmes.

In my post, I am now required to pursue an MSc but having reviewed my career options, my concerns are that I will not gain extra knowledge from the course. However, unless I have an MSc, I cannot be involved with running clinics.

This vignette is an example of the many nurses who now feel pressured to study for a higher degree to satisfy the criteria of their existing posts. However, this also illustrates a level of ambivalence towards higher academic degrees and serious doubt that non-specific clinical studies can inform senior nurses' clinical practice. The apparent practice–theory gap is indicative of a growing suspicion among some clinicians that without the acquisition of explicit performance-enhancing competences to fit them for substitution or delegated roles, this equates to no 'new knowledge'. This also suggests a resistance towards the transformational possibility of education and a denial of how the exploration of broader professional development issues and enhanced critical thinking skills can enable the practitioner to inductively grow their own knowledge of practice.

The following vignette exemplifies a converse position whereby the individual doubts their own academic credentials to fit them for the programme.

Scenario 9.2

I work as a senior practice nurse in a busy surgery in the West of Scotland and have done so for 15 years. Some of my practice patch might be described as rural. I feel that my current role is at an advanced level of practice, because it involves managing a patient case load within the practice, giving all relevant and necessary care for them, including initiating drug therapy as necessary under GP guidance and support. I also run minor illness clinics within the practice, where I am able to use my prescribing and diagnostic skills. My other role is as nurse manager for the nursing team but I am also involved in policy and strategy decision making for the whole team which includes medical colleagues. In the past 16 years my formal education and training have been developed to support my experience working in primary care. This includes courses in family planning, and diabetes care, a diploma in asthma care, and triage in the context of minor injury and illness. The last module was taken at level 3. I am now interested in pursuing an MSc but am unsure if I meet the academic criteria.

The different perspectives in Scenarios 9.1 and 9.2 might be affected by the level of specificity of each role: the first being highly focused on one client group whilst the second practitioner works with clients across the primary care sector. They both illustrate the way the practitioners migrate into new roles and then find themselves having to 'backfill' academic qualifications, in some instances for credibility, instead of seeing academic study as potentiating further role development. It further demonstrates how some practitioners might see themselves at the pinnacle of the clinical career without a vision of how they might expand their practice within that existing post and with the a view that expertise is an end point maintained solely by experience rather than new ways of thinking. This mismatch of expectation reinforces a notion, held by many clinicians and commissioners of education, that there exists a lag between workforce redesign and education provision. Thus functional training programmes are given greater spending priority, with suggestions that, in the future, professional development programmes be self-funded because they benefit the individual rather than the service.

Changes in the delivery of services

The development of new nursing roles may also be in response to advances in health technology, such as pharmacological developments, clinical interventions, implantable devices, and operative techniques (Cameron, 2000). The development of safer and minimally invasive operative procedures has created a demand, and patient expectations have also placed added pressure on service providers to offer such services. The delivery of these new advances within the climate of a reduced medical workforce has required nurses to be trained to conduct and manage clinics as part of day case surgery initiatives and under strict protocols (Royal College of Surgeons in England, 1999). In cardiac surgery too, as a result of improvements in surgical techniques and short-acting sedative drugs, the concept of fast-tracking of patients and early extubation by nurses has become established (Gale and Curry, 1999; Tripp et al., 2002). Likewise, Norton (2000) provides an account of developing a nurse-led service for weaning patients. As part of the care pathway, nurses follow protocols to warm, manage fluid and electrolyte balances, and wean patients from ventilators after open heart surgery (Scholes et al., 1999). In cases where recovery is uncomplicated, care pathways assist nurses to prepare patients for discharge home within five days and to link with a team of outreach cardiac nurses in the community to provide continuity of care. This example illustrates how nurses have filled a service niche and transferred their skills into new localities.

There are many ways in which new roles may cross professional and service boundaries (Fig. 9.1). Previously, thrombolysis has been administered only in hospitals due to the risks of intracranial bleeding, and in order to observe patients in case they develop cardiac dysrhythmias or other complications, and because of the complexity of drug administration (Albarran and

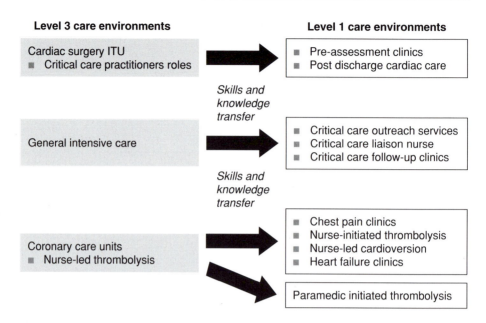

Fig. 9.1 Examples of roles transcending professional and institutional barriers.

Kapeluch, 2000). Recent advances in pharmacology have enhanced the simplicity of drug administration to a single bolus injection and improved the efficacy and safety of therapy (Leah *et al.*, 2004). Given the benefits of early administration for survival, registered paramedics are now identified as a group who can administer this treatment under a group patient directive to patients experiencing acute myocardial infarction (AMI) (National Institute for Clinical Excellence (NICE), 2002). Studies into paramedic-led thrombolysis confirm the safety of using these drugs in the pre-hospital setting (Quinn *et al.*, 1999; Keeling *et al.*, 2003; Leah *et al.*, 2004).

In another area of cardiac care, NICE (2000) has recommended that implantable cardioverter defibrillators (ICDs) should be made available to those at risk from lethal dysrhythmias or sudden cardiac death. However, Tagney (2004) identified that cardiac nurses' knowledge of ICDs was poor. Nurses were unable to give individualised information to patients about the device or how to manage lifestyle changes once discharged. Therefore, suggestions have been made to create new roles to support patients, families and other health care professionals, particularly for those based in primary care (Tagney *et al.*, 2003; Albarran *et al.*, 2004).

The development of new roles will expand and cross professional and service boundaries although this may not always be welcome (Gale and Curry, 1999; Currie, 2004; Shah and Shah, 2004). Concern has been expressed that the growing number of skills adopted by nurses may have a detrimental effect on ideas of 'caring', the nature of nursing expertise and the image of the profession (Castledine, 1995; Rushforth and Glasper, 1999; Albarran and Scholes, 2005).

Professional expectations

Professional drivers are not seen as significant in the development of new roles in nursing. However, Cameron (2000) accepts that the *Scope of Professional Practice* (UKCC, 1992a) allowed nurses to extend their skills or roles into new domains of practice. Initial areas where *Scope* enabled role expansion included defibrillation, venepuncture and weaning patients from mechanical ventilation. In some instances role expansion involved nurses in stripping of saphenous veins, suturing chests closed after open heart surgery and inserting central venous catheters; though these were unintended outcomes of *Scope* (UKCC, 1992a). In other areas, roles emerged where boundaries were blurred but where the essence of nursing remained a central element. This was common in follow-up clinics where nurses provided continuity of care and had a longitudinal perspective on care management. They were well placed to monitor patients' progress, plan interventions according to individual needs and make decisions based on clinical findings. Indeed, the *Code of Professional Practice* (UKCC, 1992b) gave nurses the right to exercise discretionary judgements on the basis that they were accountable for their actions and omissions of duty.[1] The introduction of *The Future of Professional Practice* (UKCC, 1994) set standards of practice beyond registration, particularly in relation to specialist and advanced practice. In this way practice developments were supported, and attempts to consolidate existing roles according to clinical, professional and educational benchmarks were made.

For many, the implementation of new roles was paramount to enhancing the status of the profession (Wiggens, 1998; Richardson and Cunliffe, 2003). Moreover, aside of traditional boundaries of practice being redrawn, nursing has always sought to remain dynamic and flexible and to adapt its services according to the needs of the population (Read, 1998). In its *Report on Higher Level Practice*, the UKCC (1998) recognised that the proliferation of roles and titles was confusing to the profession and did not afford the public protection. To reconcile this situation, the regulating body delineated higher levels of practice as those requiring the nurse to demonstrate autonomous practice, higher levels of decision making, improving standards of care, and developing and leading practice, and where they also made a contribution to teaching, research and supervision of staff. Rather than consolidating levels of practice by certificated or extended practices, key practice standards and academic achievement would be fulfilled (Castledine, 1998). In this way it was hoped that there would be a move away from roles embracing medical concepts,

---

[1] However, in roles that have been established as clearly defined medical substitution posts, the development and confirmation of competence are controlled by medical consultants. Practice was clearly delineated by protocols, limiting the discretionary decision making of the post-holder. These practices were considered essential for risk management to protect the post-holder, the consultant and the Trust from litigation (Vaughan, Furlong and Scholes cited in Read *et al.*, 1999).

or those considered as specialist by virtue of working in a specialist area. Furthermore, by setting specific guidelines about the domains of higher levels of practice, the Council sought to prevent others from controlling the character of nursing roles (Wiggens, 1998). However, this objective has failed to materialise due to the introduction of staffing policies which have swept away 'old-fashioned demarcations' and developed new roles to overcome medical personnel shortage (Benton, 2003; George, 2003; Albarran and Scholes, 2005). Furthermore, the Government's primary objective is 'largely focused on the transfer of tasks from highly qualified professionals to less highly qualified professionals' (NPCRD, 1999). The intention is to cut costs and to improve service efficiency (George, 2003) which bodes ill for specialist and advanced roles. Government funding via Workforce Development Confederations is focused on competency development rather than education. Short training courses are seen as the solution to manage the shortfall of qualified staff in the NHS (see below) (Thompson and Watson, 2005).

Blurring and blending of roles

Despite large numbers of students in training, there is a shortfall of nurses due to problems with recruitment and retention across all areas (Calpin-Davies and Akehurst, 1999; Rushforth and Glasper, 1999; Hall, 2002). Poor remuneration for increased responsibility, work pressures and job dissatisfaction account for the fall in available registered nurses. Attempts to improve this situation have been fostered through intraprofessional learning and shared learning of clinical skills. Also, the NHS has championed *New Ways of Working* (NHS Modernisation Agenda, 2003), job re-profiling and developing professionals with generic roles as appropriate solutions to sustain effectiveness in health service provision and meet consumer demands (Benton, 2003; Albarran and Scholes, 2005). This may be interpreted as rebalancing of deficits in technical expertise. Since nurses are the largest employee group in the NHS, they are viewed as one group whose clinical responsibilities could expand at low cost. However, this argument is flawed since it assumes there is a nursing capacity surplus (Calpin-Davies and Akehurst, 1999). The counter-argument maintains that retraining technicians and health care assistants (HCAs) to undertake tasks previously performed by nurses allows the latter to assume extra clinical duties and skills that were once the remit of doctors. *Liberating the Talents* (DH, 2002) and *New Ways of Working* (NWW) (NHS Modernisation Agency, 2003) are reactions to human resources scarcity rather than ways to influence the organisational culture. These documents imply that allowing nurses to expand their roles results in a more rewarded, fulfilled and liberated workforce. *NWW* (NHS Modernisation Agency, 2003) uses the concept of 'role redesign' to enable individuals to expand their roles and skills repertoire and break down interprofessional boundaries (Benton, 2003) to increase service options, reduce waiting times and make services more accessible (Mullally, 2004). Also, through multi-skilling and blending of professional roles and responsibilities, such workers may compensate for shortages of doctors and increase NHS capacity to treat more patients.

The discussion so far has highlighted how political, economic and professional agendas, technological advances and demographic changes within the NHS workforce have directly and indirectly influenced the development, extension and expansion of new practice roles for nurses. This is based on the assumption that there is an abundance of nurses to assume new skills and that these added responsibilities advance the profession's status. The momentum for role development has lacked vision, coordination and purpose, resulting in confusion over role boundaries, functions and standards of education. Since organisational support has not been explicit, this has fuelled uncertainty and ambiguity amongst post-holders and created difficulties in supporting individuals in the transition stages (Briggs, 1997; Lloyd Jones, 2005). Debate in this area is polarised, with some believing that role expansion benefits the profession and patient care (Rushforth and Glasper, 1999). In the current climate, there is an imperative for nurses to become more flexible and to possess a broader base of skills and knowledge. To do this, however, NHS Trusts need to devise mechanisms for supporting new roles with clear expectations over limits of professional boundaries (Levenson and Vaughan, 1999). Therefore, rigorous evaluation of the new roles, with a focus on patient and organisational outcomes, is imperative (Rushforth and Glasper, 1999; Thompson and Stewart, 2002; Mullally, 2004).

The nature and scope of nursing roles

In this next section the nature and diversity of contemporary practice roles are analysed. Roles are mapped out on a continuum with substitution of tasks at one end and autonomous practice at the other (Fig. 9.2). In each case, the scope and contribution of each role are examined alongside the implications for individuals, the profession and patients. This classification focuses on role characteristics and activity and is designed to reflect on current and emerging roles within critical care nursing.

For simplicity 'nurse-led' is used to capture the essence, domain and functions associated with a variety of roles in nursing practice that are pre-fixed in this way. Although 'nurse-led' is not sufficiently defined in the literature, its use incorporates a range of services delivered by specialist nurses, nurse practitioners and nurse consultants (Briggs, 1997; Corner, 2002). Nurse-led posts have evolved to manage acute and chronic conditions, and to provide continuity, co-ordination and more personalised services to patients, especially where there are shortages in the medical workforce (Scholes *et al.*, 1999; Cullum *et al.*, 2005). The spectrum of nurse-led roles in critical care are characterised as substitution for medical tasks that are governed by protocols and undertaken within the organisation of current service delivery, rather than having an explicit managerial orientation (Richardson and Cunliffe, 2003; Cullum *et al.*, 2005).

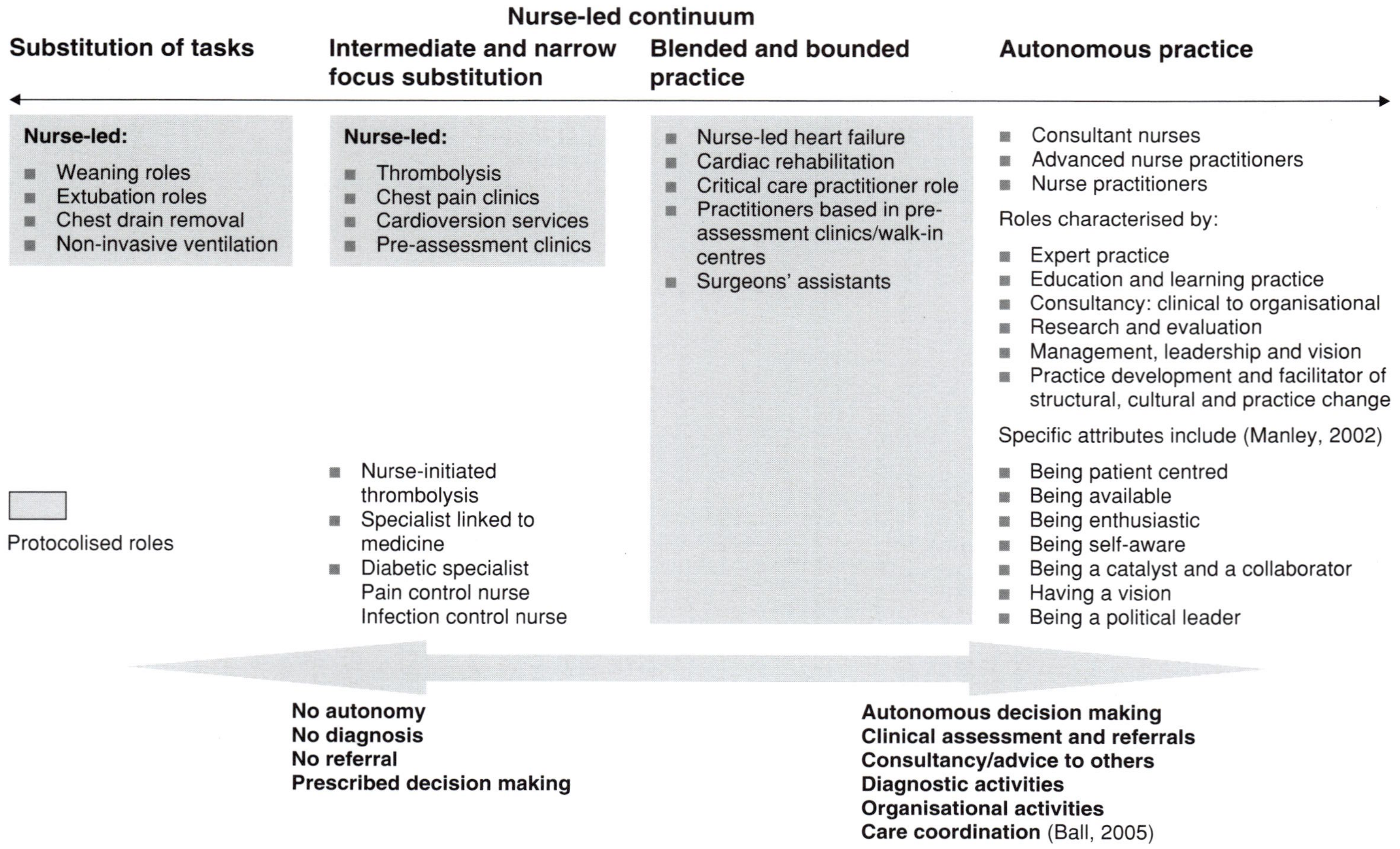

Nurse-led continuum

Substitution of tasks	Intermediate and narrow focus substitution	Blended and bounded practice	Autonomous practice
Nurse-led: ■ Weaning roles ■ Extubation roles ■ Chest drain removal ■ Non-invasive ventilation	**Nurse-led:** ■ Thrombolysis ■ Chest pain clinics ■ Cardioversion services ■ Pre-assessment clinics	■ Nurse-led heart failure ■ Cardiac rehabilitation ■ Critical care practitioner role ■ Practitioners based in pre-assessment clinics/walk-in centres ■ Surgeons' assistants	■ Consultant nurses ■ Advanced nurse practitioners ■ Nurse practitioners Roles characterised by: ■ Expert practice ■ Education and learning practice ■ Consultancy: clinical to organisational ■ Research and evaluation ■ Management, leadership and vision ■ Practice development and facilitator of structural, cultural and practice change Specific attributes include (Manley, 2002) ■ Being patient centred ■ Being available ■ Being enthusiastic ■ Being self-aware ■ Being a catalyst and a collaborator ■ Having a vision ■ Being a political leader

■ Nurse-initiated thrombolysis
■ Specialist linked to medicine
■ Diabetic specialist
■ Pain control nurse
■ Infection control nurse

Protocolised roles

No autonomy
No diagnosis
No referral
Prescribed decision making

Autonomous decision making
Clinical assessment and referrals
Consultancy/advice to others
Diagnostic activities
Organisational activities
Care coordination (Ball, 2005)

Fig. 9.2 Continuum and characteristics of nurse-led roles.

Substitution of tasks

Previously nurses doing medical tasks such as obtaining intravenous access, defibrillation, wound suturing and recording a 12-lead electrocardiogram (ECG) were required to undergo additional training and certification as these tasks were role extensions. Due to increased demands for health care, nurses now assume a wider set of clinical skills including the insertion of central lines, nurse-led extubation/weaning and nurse-led chest-drain removal (Hamilton *et al.*, 1995; Gale and Curry, 1999; Christensen, 2002). The justification for accepting these responsibilities into nursing work is in part due to political expediency. Practical reasons such as early patient transfer to wards are also cited as explaining the need for nurses to undertake medical functions (Christensen, 2002). Protocols or guidelines are used to regulate staff actions, with the aim of minimising patient risk. Nurses have no freedom to make decisions outside the protocol without first referring to doctors. Generally, nurses who meet specific unit criteria, for example seniority of grade, are eligible to expand their duties (Christiansen, 2002). Since task substituted roles are based on episodic interactions, and seen as low risk, there is the potential for fragmenting care, particularly if delegated to junior staff (Richardson and Cunliffe, 2003). Application protocols place restrictions on the scope of practice, and as such the risk to the post-holder, consultant and Trust is reduced. Such roles enhance the care of patients and reduce delays in treatment but do little to augment the professional career of nurses.

Intermediate and narrow-focus substitution

In these posts, the level of medical substitution involves more technical activities. The literature defines nurse-led or nurse-directed as being involved with shifting professional boundaries and working in partnership with medical staff (Thompson and Stewart, 2002; Richardson and Cunliffe, 2003). Nurse-led thrombolysis post-holders are experienced coronary care nurses who conduct clinical patient examinations and interpret and diagnose ECGs, but who refer to medical staff to prescribe treatment or other interventions (Smallwood, 2004). Individuals are based in one setting and they perform medical functions to streamline service organisation. Their actions are directed by protocols and patient group directives. Training and close supervision by doctors may be provided but ultimately the focus of care is narrow. Furthermore, in some instances, post-holders are required by their medical colleagues to abandon their title 'nurse' in favour of the term 'practitioner' to reflect their redefined medical substitution role (Scholes *et al.*, 1999).

The introduction of nurse-led cardioversion services is one example (Quinn, 1998; Currie *et al.*, 2004). The rationale for change here arose because of ineffective use of coronary care beds, limited availability of medical staff and recognition that patient care was sub-optimal. Cardioversion services were implemented following a period in which post-holders received supervised training and achieved locally agreed competencies in advanced life support and protocol use. These two initiatives exemplify the substitution of medical tasks, a narrow focus of care, intermittent nurse–patient interactions and restricted autonomy. Nurse-led does not signify that other health care professionals or doctors are excluded from the actual management of patients' care (Albarran, 2005): in both the above projects anaesthetists were available. Nurse-led services function differently in community settings where post-holders may provide some treatments, consultations and health information (Cullum *et al.*, 2005).

A second example is that of nurse-initiated thrombolysis, whereby nurses have authority to start treatments without referring to medical staff, but their practice is bounded by protocols and patient group directives (Albarran, 2004). Most of these posts are described as 'innovative' and 'effective' based on audits comparing the effectiveness of nurses' intervention with those performed by junior or middle-level doctors (ibid.). Their effectiveness is enhanced because of the economic and patient benefits that accrue as nurses have assumed key roles to meet government standards. However, the criteria for appointing post-holders are idiosyncratic, random or based on physician preferences.

Table 9.1 A comparison in features and activities between intermediate and narrow focus substitution roles and autonomous practice roles.

Intermediate and narrow focus substitution

- Appointments may be based on local criteria or individuals may be selected because of their skills and knowledge
- Academic qualifications not essential
- Assessment is medically driven
- Referrals are based on protocol
- Ability to request additional tests or initiate interventions must be in consultation with a doctor
- Prescribing must follow patient group directives
- Decision making is bound within protocols
- Limited scope for expanding role
- Approach to care is centred on achievement of tasks
- Relationship with patients is of a short and episodic nature

Autonomous practice (e.g. nurse practitioners, consultant nurses)

- Appointments are through meeting specified criteria, expert practice is central
- First degree or Master's level qualification is essential
- Initiates clinical assessment
- Can refer patients to relevant agencies
- Can request additional investigations independently
- Has prescribing rights
- Independent decision making
- Opportunity to expand practice and personal development
- Integrated and holistic approach to care
- Relationship with patients may be of a lasting nature
- There is a collegiate relationship with members of the inter-disciplinary team

With regard to preparing nurses to administer thrombolysis, there are disparities in programme content, delivery modes and competency assessments (Albarran, 2004). This type of work essentially replicates medically based duties; practice is protocol driven with little opportunity for holistic care. Table 9.1 highlights some of the core characteristics of narrow focus/intermediate substitution roles.

In the vignette below, some of the dilemmas associated with moving into intermediate substitution roles are illustrated. The partnership between nursing and medicine in managing shifting professional boundaries is demonstrated by the Trust agreeing to train and equip this nurse to function in a dedicated sphere of cardiology. However, problems arose because the focus of care was medically driven, and because the Trust created this post to address national targets set out by the Department of Health (DH, 2000a). As a consequence, there was little opportunity for the post-holder to influence the delivery of care in a meaningful way and this created a 'glass ceiling effect' (Levenson and Vaughan, 1999) which hindered career progression. The excessive reliance on clinical protocols became a barrier for the post-holder to exercise clinical discretion and make autonomous judgements.

Scenario 9.3

I trained in Northern Ireland as a RN + BSc (Hons). I really enjoyed my training and after qualifying I moved to London to get some clinical experience. After two years I travelled and did a year abroad working in a very busy and dynamic CCU.

When I got back to the UK, I took up a post as an E grade and within six months I was appointed as an F grade. I also enrolled on a distance learning MSc in nursing practice.

In my practice, an opportunity to work as a part-time sister and as a clinical trials co-ordinator became available and I was successful in securing the post. Initially, the combination of roles gave me a lot and I was able to expand different skills and take on new challenges. However, after two and a half years, I felt I needed a change and the medical consultant and lead sister advised me that the Trust was planning to open an acute chest pain admission clinic.

Although I had an MSc, this had not given me the skills I needed. Subsequently I enrolled at the local university and undertook M level modules in history taking, examination skills and diagnostic reasoning. Prior to the new unit opening, I received a lot of support and extra training from senior medical staff in ECG interpretation, differential diagnosis, interpreting basic x-rays, etc. It was also great to have the experience in designing protocols and visiting other centres. I have now been in post for four months and realise that I cannot continue in it forever. I can't see myself being challenged in this role for much longer. I will probably give it another 6 months. I am thinking of studying medicine as I am only 29 years of age.

Scholes *et al.* (1999) cautioned that in some cases roles can become so focused upon medical duties that the post-holders feel they no longer practise nursing and are led to consider the merits of maintaining their nursing registration. In the example in Scenario 9.3, the post-holder clearly identified how her role has channelled her toward a medical career rather than back into a senior nursing role. Viewing this through a 'skills escalator lens', such transition would be viewed favourably. However, viewing this through a 'retention of expertise lens', one can question the merits of such an approach, especially when considering the level of training and investment already devoted to the development of this practitioner relative to their length of stay in post.

The ad hoc inception, preparation and evaluation of new roles has gathered pace in response to the demand for new people to work differently (see Chapter 2.) As a consequence little consideration is given to how these roles might fit into existing professional career structures or how individuals may progress after holding such posts (Levenson and Vaughan, 1999; Albarran, 2004). Therefore, new incumbents might well be highly excited by the prospects and challenges of assuming such roles only to find themselves in a potential career cul-de-sac. This is made even more precarious for those assuming roles on temporary contracts, especially if the role has been classified as having 'pilot status' (Scholes *et al.*, 1999). In such situations it is expedient for practitioners to reflect upon the tasks they might be required to perform and seek to enhance rather than exclusively replace their professional skills repertoire. This can be a difficult task when exposed to the full weight of medical socialisation when in role (Vaughan, Furlong and Scholes cited in Read *et al.*, 1999).

Corner (2002) and others have identified practical difficulties in relation to the training and supervision of nurses assuming responsibility for aspects of medical practice. Medical training has involved close and structured supervision of students in their practice but such opportunities may not be automatically available to nurses (Rosen and Mountford, 2002). Albarran (2004) identified that the lack of uniform appointment criteria for nurses in dedicated cardiac posts and the extreme variation in levels of training and supervision offered by medical staff left some nurses feeling anxious about the added duties for which they had not been formally prepared. Decisions over the minimum educational preparation for new roles and who determines practice competences are issues rarely debated outside the orbit of the team involved in the generation of the new role. This can place the practitioner in an extremely vulnerable position, especially where lines of responsibility are blurred or made obtuse by cross-professional working.

Blended and bounded roles

In blended roles some elements of post-holders' practice are based on medical functions but these have been integrated into a nursing model of care. They might provide a series of services, previously outside their professional remit, which enhance the co-ordination of care and continuity of service and provide sustained consultations. With blended roles, nurses may establish stronger continuity and rapport with patients and their families. Since the demand for doctors' skills has increased, nurses have acquired new skills to respond to the ongoing changes. These posts can be regarded as complementary to medicine rather than adversarial as can happen with intermediate substitution of roles (Scholes *et al.*, 1999; Shah and Shah, 2004). There is a discreet level of autonomy, and post-holders exercise judgements without always referring to protocols. In cardiac rehabilitation and heart failure, post-holders may have multiple responsibilities including coordinating care, teaching, counselling and coaching, depending on the patient's stage of recovery (Fridlund, 2002; Strömberg, 2002). Post-holders need to be knowledgeable and experienced, have advanced interpersonal skills and be competent to work independently to undertake delegated activities, namely titrating medications, adjusting patient goals and negotiating targets based on assessments and protocols. These roles also support patients through various stages of transition, for example from hospital to home to continue rehabilitation. The nature of nurse–patient interaction is likely to be sustained over a long period. These posts bring added value to patient interactions which are reflected by the clinical expertise, knowledge and skills of the post-holders.

Physicians' assistant (PA) roles were introduced to substitute nurses[2] for junior hospital doctors to perform basic surgical procedures such as harvesting saphenous veins and closing surgical wounds. These roles are about improving throughput of patients and reducing waiting lists. PAs have a 'delegated' scope to perform duties and provide care for patients under supervision of a physician. These assistants will have undergone intensive surgical/medical training. They can also conduct physical assessments and order clinical investigations but there is concern that their practice will not include nursing values. The roles are clearly bounded within a medical model, and although they are expanding the boundaries of the profession, this is being achieved by the medicalisation of nursing roles. However, to their credit many post-holders have shaped their duties to focus on providing continuity of patient care by adopting a more holistic outlook (Boss, 2002; Knight, 2003). For Knight (2003) the unique relationship that PAs have with patients and the use of specially developed skills allow them to make informed decisions about patients in their care. Bowey and Caballero (1996) described one role which combined responsibility for laparoscopic procedures and managing a caseload of patients who were admitted and discharged on agreed protocols. While roles which combine nursing and medical elements may help to overcome workforce depletion and benefit patients, they do not necessarily advance nursing practice (Manley, 1996) as they do not promote the values of the profession.

---

[2] It is recognised that these roles may be assumed by health care workers other than nurses, and that in the future direct entry into Physicians' Assistant training is likely.

So far the concept of blended and bounded roles has been presented as a way of distinguishing between the substitution of medical activities and adapting such responsibilities and embracing them within a nursing framework. Whether they are effective, are accepted by patients and are seen as a necessity is yet to be determined. However, they may be used to manage the shortfall of health care staff and suppress professional autonomy. The implementation of 'blended posts' could be interpreted as an attempt to make role expansion more acceptable professionally and avoid focusing the debate on occupational blurring of roles. Blended roles may meet the demands of the NHS, not only because the skills pool increases, but also because there is a ready-made and responsive workforce which may be deployed across the sector to work efficiently and effectively. Within this approach, nursing functions such as health promotion, physical evaluation, psychosocial management and leadership skills can be merged with doctors' roles such as conducting clinical assessments, and treating and discharging patients. However, the repackaging of blended roles conceals the increased responsibilities that will be expected of nurses, and implementation may erode nursing's image and identity. Blending of roles may mean more than restructuring, retooling and redesigning the whole approach to patient care: it may have an impact on the intraprofessional agenda.

Examples of autonomous practice

Nurse practitioners
The nurse practitioner (NP) is a relatively new role in the UK. It has become well defined in terms of national and international criteria that include a focus on client-centred practice (Carlisle, 2005). NPs were forced to reinvent themselves due to debates and disagreements about their scope of practice, and about the blurring of role boundaries which were considered to be about expanding primary medical practice and reducing general practitioners' workload (Albarran and Whittle, 1999; Furlong and Smith, 2005). Another view was that NPs were registered nurses prepared for the purpose of improving health assessment, managing the delivery of patient services in the community and medicalising nursing practice (Castledine, 1995). The role of NP generated much debate in the nursing press. A universal definition of NPs and advanced nurse practitioners (ANPs) was developed (Carlisle, 2005) as a result of the rise in their number, uncertainty about the essential clinical and educational criteria for the role, their benefits to the image of the profession, and concerns about them promoting a medicalised model of care.

Nurse consultants
The role of the consultant nurse is multidimensional and integrates a number of components working synergistically to advance nursing rather than medical practice (Manley, 2002). Unlike other roles, consultant nurses have a clinical remit of 'diagnostic' and 'organisational' responsibilities (Ball, 2005)

and are accorded the same status as medical consultants (Waller, 1998). The NHS Executive (1998) also expected that these individuals should be educated to masters level or beyond.

Nurse consultants have an explicit role to foster leadership, clinical expertise, teaching and research responsibilities.

Consequences of new nursing roles

Over the past three decades there have been a number of concerns which have plagued the profession in respect of the emergence of new roles. These are issues that pertain to the dilution of knowledge, the use of health care assistants (see Chapter 8), tensions over the preparation of advanced practice and ways of enabling role transition.

Loss of experiential wisdom

Developing new nursing posts such as critical care outreach programmes not only involves the loss of expert practitioners and role models from intensive care units but also depletes knowledge levels. Over a period of time, although the knowledge base and expertise of nurses in high acuity areas (level 1 environments) increase and benefit the care of patients, they may potentially decline in level 3 areas. While sharing of skills, knowledge and expertise is vital in developing the care of patients in acuity areas, this must be balanced with maintaining and advancing nursing expertise in critical settings. It may be speculated that, where once nurses had a broad level of understanding, for example about diabetes and pain management, this has decreased due to specialist nursing roles. Because of their additional training, education and position within an organisation, specialist nurses are viewed as being in possession of detailed subject knowledge and expertise. They are called upon to review and advise on the care of patients' individual and complex needs. It may be reasoned that the motivation to develop knowledge, skill or expertise in managing infection, nutrition or pain control becomes a personal choice and not a mandatory activity. The net effect of this is that the overall knowledge base amongst ward staff is diluted and nurses trust that those who have specialist roles or who are in outreach positions will resolve their care of patients with specialist medical needs and simultaneously be a source of knowledge or advice.

Within medical circles, there is also a sense of crisis about allowing nurses and other health care workers to undertake aspects of their work which were vital to junior doctor training (Bridges, 2004; Latimer, 2004). The growth of multidisciplinary teams has resulted in a more collaborative model of decision making and an increased willingness to share skills and roles (Read, 1998). Doctors may experience uneasiness that they no longer hold the power base in decisions about patient care, because currently it *is* interdisciplinary teams that deliver modern health care (Benger and Hoskins, 2005). There are shared concerns about the impact of new roles on medicine and nursing, in terms of training, remuneration and occupational objectives. Furthermore, by embracing former medical duties, nurses reinvent themselves as handmaidens to medicine and pass nursing care to others (Rushford and Glasper, 1999). However, new roles and role expansion provide nurses with opportunities for full team working and delivering comprehensive care. In many instances they are formally developing their clinical assessment and diagnostic reasoning skills. The challenge is to create roles that integrate new skills and knowledge relevant to each of the health care disciplines but which retain a set of patient-centred focus core values for each profession. To do this there need to be coherence and national standards about appointment criteria and responsibilities of new critical care roles that link with *Agenda for Change* (DH, 1999b). Evidence is required that explores the impact of these roles on care delivery and on health care services and not solely on financial measures (Cullum *et al.*, 2005).

Educational preparation and advanced roles

Over the years there has been intense debate about the level of educational preparation for nurse practitioners, advanced nurse practitioners, consultant nurses and other titles (Ball, 1997, 1999; Rolfe and Fulbrook, 1998; Albarran and Whittle, 1999). Like many countries, few have protected titles, regulated standards of entry, and standardised educational pathways as means to distinguish such roles. In the UK, a satisfactory solution has failed to materialise because the UKCC remained silent about the type of preparation or qualifications required for nursing roles beyond registration. In 1994, the Council identified that specialist practice required the minimum of a degree qualification (UKCC, 1994). This led to mass preoccupation among nurses with their academic standing in terms of accreditation. The other difficulty has been that courses in the UK have not been suitable or sufficiently relevant to support clinical and theoretical expectations of nurses working as advanced nurse practitioners and consultant nurses. Limited opportunities for interdisciplinary learning are other criticisms. Recent discussions emphasise the emerging global agreement that educational preparation for NP, ANP and consultant nurse posts should be at masters level and focus on advancing practice, improving health services and acquisition of leadership and innovation skills (NHS Executive, 1998; ICN, 2002; Carlisle, 2005). This is in line with North America where such roles have a long history (Albarran and Whittle, 1999; RCN, 2004). The Nursing and Midwifery Council has recently started consultation on a framework for standards for post-registration nursing to take account of national and international developments (NMC, 2004). This is an attempt to consolidate the myriad of posts that reflect higher-level practice. By assimilating the international guidelines the NMC will be setting coherent and unambiguous standards about how to achieve a recordable qualification and so protect the public.

Moving role transition forwards – facilitators and barriers

A major theme in the 21st century is identifying how nurses can become effective in their new roles and make a positive difference to patient outcomes and health care delivery. Nurses will be instrumental to service development and delivery, and the challenge facing employers is to facilitate a smooth role transition by supporting individuals in their adjustment.

There are many factors which influence role transition (Glen and Waddington, 1998):

- role requirements;
- induction and socialisation processes;
- prior occupational socialisation;
- individual/personality and characteristics.

Manley (2002) argues that personal attributes and qualities such as being available and patient-centred, being a change agent and a catalyst for innovation, being a collaborator and having a vision and the ability to negotiate by political astuteness are fundamental to the effectiveness of consultant nurse roles (see Table 9.1) and explain their success. Role transition can also be facilitated by defining the population health needs and involving key stakeholders affected to promote a shared understanding of post-holder responsibilities (Bryant-Lukosius and DiCenso, 2004). However, Ball (1999) and Lloyd Jones's (2005) recent meta-synthesis emphasise post-holder confidence. Without this, the role might not be seen as relevant to the profession. Other skills identified include political astuteness, ability to manage conflict, stamina, and promoting self (Ball, 1999; Lloyd Jones, 2005).

Organisational culture has an impact too. Having clear definitions of role boundaries and professional autonomy are essential features of these posts if they are to be successful (Bamford and Gibson, 1999; Lloyd Jones, 2005). By providing training and staff opportunities to develop people in their roles and ensure that they share experiences; by formulating career pathways; and by providing supervision to support post-holders in their new positions, organisations are also likely to be successful in facilitating role transition (Bamford and Gibson, 1999; Lloyd Jones, 2005). The socialisation of new roles into an organisation needs to be a gradual process and it should enable the incumbents to develop networks, appreciate the demands of the job and understand organisational culture and structure (Glen and Waddington, 1998). Scholes *et al.* (1999) report that post-holders working in such institutions tend to remain in role for a number of years as a result of strong collegiate support and the enabling organisational infrastructure.

A study of the first 153 consultant nurses identified that 50% were appointed from within their own Trust (Guest *et al.*, 2001), strongly suggesting organisational investment in preparing nurses for senior clinical posts. Ball (1999) and Lloyd Jones (2005) identify having prior clinical experience and credibility as additional elements supporting effective integration. Working within the same Trust and using 'insider intelligence' facilitate role transition because individuals know how the organisation functions and are aware of service delivery issues.

Yet, despite this, many consultant nurses and others who operate at similar levels encounter role ambiguity, role conflict, work overload and problems with role boundaries and autonomy, which may act as barriers to role transition (Guest *et al.*, 2001; Lloyd Jones, 2005). Regardless of insider intelligence, an absence of established networks, lack of a mentor or supervisor, and an inability to practise autonomously to define personal objectives and priorities and to implement change can all impact on successful role transition (Glen and Waddington, 1998). Previously, Albarran and Whittle (1999) reported that integration dilemmas for nurses performing at these levels remained unresolved within the profession. It might be that these innovative roles challenge accepted orthodoxies about the nature of nursing and that post-holders are viewed with hostility and resentment, and experience professional isolation and lack of peer endorsement. However, Guest *et al.* (2001) and Lloyd Jones (2005) have identified that individuals with high levels of organisational commitment, effective intraprofessional relationships and peer support experienced less resistance and were therefore more effective. Almost all consultants believed that their role improved quality of patient care and career opportunities; 70% believed such posts helped to retain experienced staff. At a personal level, 82% reported high levels of professional commitment, 84% felt the job provided personal growth and development opportunities, 50% claimed the post lived up to their expectations and 35% stated high levels of reward fairness (Guest *et al.*, 2001). Managing role transition and nurturing clinical expertise are components that need wider debate within the profession. Although it is an area of great complexity, research is needed that explores the most effective way to support practitioners.

Conclusion

In the past three decades there has been an explosion of new roles, primarily driven by political and economic forces outside nursing. The evolution of new roles has been ad hoc and haphazard. Nursing has not been clear about the type of education and training that new roles may require and has prevaricated about opportunities for career development, defining role boundaries and the need to assess competence. The typology of roles over the wide diversity of posts available reflects the confusion that exists. These issues apply to critical care where countless nurse-led initiatives have emerged in disparate fashion. Collectively these factors have had a negative effect on the transition of many roles and have limited the effectiveness of nurses.

Although nursing has been slow to agree educational profiles, there now seems to be a consensus that nurses working at an NP or nurse consultant level are required to be educated to masters level. Beyond this, there needs to be a systematic and rational approach to enable nurses to progress on the basis of skills, experience and academic achievements. Preparation should include clinical and professional competencies as well as developing personal qualities and attributes. There also needs to be flexibility in the preparation of individuals, and recognition that few will reach the highest levels of practice. Opportunities should be available for nurses to craft their personal journey in a way that enables them to mature professionally and intellectually. Nursing needs to critically evaluate whether patient care and the organisation of service delivery are enhanced by nurses extending or expanding their roles. Also, the repercussion from these changes needs to be considered: for example, whether the quality of nursing care is adversely affected as HCAs extend and expand their role.

The current government is committed to reforming the health service and dismantling occupational boundaries which in the past have stifled innovation and improvements. If nurses are adopting new roles and ways of working, then they might consider how nursing values and philosophies of care could be integrated. The nursing profession needs to be shrewd to manage tensions over role ambiguity and uncertainty about role boundaries. Standards that will support staff during role transition are needed so they may make a lasting impact on the delivery of nursing care and respond to future challenge in new and imaginative ways. Research has identified the impact of specific nursing roles on the quality of care, but there is still insufficient evidence on the structure and processes of care, the factors that improve care, whether care is cost-effective when delivered by different health care providers and the overall effect of role substitution on patient experiences and outcomes.

In the next chapter future challenges that face the provision of critical care services are explored to identify the macroprofessional learning transitions that will be needed to meet the needs of patients and their relatives.

Acknowledgement

I would like to thank Dr David Pontin, University of the West of England, for his valuable critical comments and editing skills.

References

Albarran JW (2004) Preparing nurses to initiate thrombolytic therapy for patients with an acute myocardial infarction – is there a consensus? *Nurse Education in Practice* 4(1): 60–68.

Albarran JW (2005) Nurse-led care-definitions. *British Medical Journal* (rapid response). http://bmj.bmjjournals.com/cgi/content/extract/330/7493/682.

Albarran JW and Fulbrook P (1998) Advanced nursing practice: a historical perspective. In: Fulbrook P. and Rolfe G. (eds). *Perspectives on Advanced Nursing*. Oxford: Butterworth Heinemann.

Albarran JW and Kapeluch H (2000) Role of the nurse in thrombolysis – expanding the clinical horizons. In: Cruikshank JP, Bradbury M. and Ashurst S (eds). *Aspects in Cardiovascular Nursing*. Salisbury: Quay Publications, Mark Allen Publishing.

Albarran JW and Scholes J (2005) Blurred, blended or disappearing – the image of critical care nursing. *Nursing in Critical Care* **10**(1): 2–4.

Albarran JW and Whittle C (1999) Specialist and advanced practice: the debates. In: Littlewood J (ed.). *Current Issues in Community Nursing: Specialist Practice in Primary Healthcare*. Edinburgh: Churchill Livingstone.

Albarran JW, Tagney J and James J (2004) Partners of ICD patients – an exploratory study of their experiences. *European Journal of Cardiovascular Nursing* **3**(3): 201–210.

Ball C (1997) Planning for the future: advanced nursing practice in critical care. *Intensive and Critical Care Nursing* **13**: 17–25.

Ball C (1999) Revealing higher levels of nursing practice. *Intensive and Critical Care Nursing* **15**: 65–76.

Ball J (2005) *Maxi Nurses – Advanced and Specialist Nursing Roles. Results from a Survey of RCN Members in Advanced and Specialist Nursing Roles*. London: RCN.

Ball J and Pike G (2005) *Managing to Work Differently: Results from the RCN Employment Survey 2005*. London: RCN.

Bamford O and Gibson F (1999) The clinical nurse specialist role: development strategies that facilitate role evolution. *Advancing Clinical Nursing* **3**(4): 143–151.

Benger J and Hoskins R (2005) Nurses are autonomous healthcare professionals delivering expert care. *British Medical Journal* **330**: 1084.

Benner P (1984) *From Novice to Expert: Excellence and Power in Clinical Nursing*. Mento Park, CA: Addison Wesley.

Benton D (2003) Agenda for change: the knowledge and skills framework. *Nursing Standard* **18**(6): 33–39.

Blue L, Lang E, McMurray JJV, Davie AP, McDonough TA, Mardoch DR *et al.* (2001) Randomised controlled trial of specialist nurse interventions for heart failure. *British Medical Journal* **323**: 715–718.

Boss S (2002) Expanding the perioperative role: the surgeon's assistant. *British Journal of Perioperative Nursing* **12**(3): 105, 107–109, 111–113.

Bowey D and Caballero C (1996) A lead role. *Nursing Times* **92**(30): 29–31.

Bridges J (2004) Training repercussions. *British Medical Journal* **329**: 892–894.

Briggs M (1997) Developing nursing roles. *Nursing Standard* **11**(36): 49–55.

Brown R (1995) The politics of specialist/advanced practice conflict or confusion? *British Journal of Nursing* **4**(16): 944–948.

Bryant-Lukosius D and DiCenso A (2004) A framework for the introduction and evaluation of advanced roles. *Journal of Advanced Nursing* **48**(5): 530–540.

Calpin-Davies P and Akehurst R (1999) Doctor–nurse substitution: the workforce equation. *Journal of Nursing Management* **7**: 71–79.

Cameron A (2000) New role developments in context. In: Humphris D and Masterson A (eds). *Developing New Clinical Roles*. Edinburgh: Churchill Livingstone.

Carlisle D (2005) New nursing roles: deciding the future for Scotland, www.scotland.gov.uk/library5/health/nnrdf-05.asp (accessed 11 February 2005).

Castledine G (1995) Will the nurse practitioner be a mini-doctor or a maxi-nurse? *British Journal of Nursing* **4**(16): 938–939.

Castledine G (1998) From specialist practice role to level of practice. *British Journal of Nursing* **7**(11): 682.

Christensen M (2002) Nurse-led chest drain removal in a cardiac high dependency unit. *Nursing in Critical Care* **7**(2): 67–72.

Cline CMJ, Israelsson BYA, Willenheimer RB, Broms K and Erhardt LR (1998) Cost effective management programme for heart failure reduces hospitalisation. *Heart* **80**: 442–446.

Coad S and Haines S (1999) Supporting staff caring for acutely ill patients in acute care areas. *Nursing in Critical Care* **4**: 245–248.

Coombs M and Dillon A (2002) Crossing boundaries, redefining care: the role of the critical care outreach team. *Journal of Clinical Nursing* **11**(3): 387–393.

Corner J (2002) The role of nurse-led care in cancer management. *The Lancet Oncology* **4**(10): 631–636.

Cullum N, Spilsbury K and Richardson G (2005) Editorial: Nurse-led care. *British Medical Journal* **330**: 682–683.

Currie GP (2004) Maintaining common sense and junior doctor skills. *British Medical Journal* **329**: 892–894.

Currie MP, Karwatowski P, Perera J and Langford E (2004) Introduction of a nurse led DC cardioversion service in a day surgery unit: prospective audit. *British Medical Journal* **329**: 892–894.

Cuthbertson CH (2003) Critical care outreach – cash for no questions. *British Journal of Anaesthesia* **90**(1): 5–6.

Department of Health (1997) *The New NHS: Modern and Dependable.* London: The Stationery Office.

Department of Health (1998) *A First Class Service: Quality in the New NHS.* London: The Stationery Office.

Department of Health (1999a) *Making a Difference: Strengthening the Nursing, Midwifery, Health Visiting Contribution to Health and Healthcare.* London: The Stationery Office.

Department of Health (1999b) *Agenda for Change: Modernising the NHS Pay System.* London: The Stationery Office. www.info.doh.gov.uk/doh/coin4.nsf/page/ HSC-1999-035?OpenDocument (accessed 27 September 2005).

Department of Health (2000a) *National Service Framework for Coronary Heart Disease.* London: The Stationery Office.

Department of Health (2000b) *The NHS Plan: a Plan for Investment, a Plan for Reform.* London: The Stationery Office.

Department of Health (2000c) *Comprehensive Critical Care: A Review of Adult Critical Care Services,* London: DH.

Department of Health (2002) *Liberating the Talents: Helping Primary Care Trusts to Deliver the NHS Plan.* London: The Stationery Office.

Department of Health (2005) Arrhythmias and sudden cardiac death. In: *National Service Framework for Coronary Heart Disease.* London: The Stationery Office.

Doyal L, Dowling S and Cameron A (1998) *Challenging Practice: an Evaluation of Four Innovatory Posts in the South-West.* Bristol: Policy Press.

Fridlund B (2002) The role of the nurse in cardiac rehabilitation programmes. *European Journal of Cardiovascular Nursing* **1**(1): 15–18.

Furlong E and Smith R (2005) Advanced nursing practice: policy, education and role development. *Journal of Advanced Nursing* **14**: 1059–1066.

Gale C and Curry S (1999) Evidencing nurse-led accelerated extubation post-cardiac surgery. *Nursing in Critical Care* **4**(4): 165–170.

Garrard C and Young JD (1998) Sub-optimal care of patients before admission to intensive care. *British Medical Journal* **316**: 1841–1842.

George G (2003) Agenda for change. www.labournet.net/ukunion/0302/afc1.html (accessed 27 September 2005).

Gibson F and Bamford O (2001) Focus group interviews to examine the role and development of the clinical nurse specialist. *Journal of Nursing Management* 9: 331–342.

Glen S and Waddington S (1998) Role transition from staff nurse to clinical nurse specialist: a case study. *Journal of Clinical Nursing* 7: 283–290.

Goldhill DR, Singh SR, Tarling MM, Worthington L, Mulcahy A, White S *et al.* (1998) The patient at risk team: identifying and managing critically ill ward patients. *British Journal of Anaesthesia* 1998 **81**: 812P.

Guest D, Redfern S, Wilson-Barnett J, Dewe P, Peccei R, Rosenthal P, *et al.* (2001) *A Preliminary Evaluation of the Establishment of the Nurse, Midwife and Health Visitor Consultants: A report to the Department of Health.* London: Kings College London.

Hall R (2002) Fifth report on the provision of services for patients with heart disease. *Heart* **88** (Suppl. III): iii1–iii59.

Hamilton H, O'Byrne M and Nicholai L (1995) Central lines inserted by clinical nurse specialists. *Nursing Times* **91**(17): 38–39.

International Council of Nurses (2002) ICN announces its position on advanced nursing roles. *International Nursing Review* **49**: 199–206.

Keeling P, Hughes D, Price L, Shaw S and Barton A (2003) Safety and feasibility of prehospital thrombolysis carried out by paramedics. *British Medical Journal* **327**: 27–28.

Knight G (2003) Nurse-led discharge from high dependency unit. *Nursing in Critical Care* **8**(2): 56–61.

Latimer MD (2004) Medical training implications. *British Medical Journal* **329**: 892–894.

Leah V, Clark C, Doyle K and Coats T (2004) Does a single bolus thrombolytic reduce door to needle time in a district general hospital? *Emergency Medicine Journal* **21**(2): 162–164.

Levenson R and Vaughan B (1999) *Developing New Roles in Practice: a Research-based Approach.* London: King's Fund.

Lloyd Jones M (2005) Role development and effective practice in specialist and advanced practice roles in acute hospital settings: a systematic review and meta-synthesis. *Journal of Advanced Nursing* 49(2): 191–209.

Manley K (1996) Advanced practice is not about medicalising nursing roles. *Nursing in Critical Care* **1**(2): 56–57.

Manley K (2002) Refining the consultant nurse framework: commentary on critique. *Nursing in Critical Care* **7**(2): 84–87.

Martins JL, Fox KF, Wood DA, Lefroy DC, Collier TJ and Peters NS (2004) Rapid access arrhythmia clinic for the diagnosis and management of new arrhythmias presenting in the community: a prospective, descriptive study. *Heart* **90**: 877–881.

Morgan RJM, Williams F and Wright MM (1997) An early warning scoring system for detecting developing critical illness. *Clinical Intensive Care* **8**: 100.

Mullally S (2004) Extending the nursing role, themed HTA update. http://www.ncchta.org/news/index.htm#Update (accessed 17 April 2005).

Murch P and Warren K (2001) Developing the role of critical care liaison nurse. *Nursing in Critical Care* **6**(5): 221–225.

Murray C, Read S and McCabe C (1995) *Reduction in Junior Doctors' Hours: the Nursing Contribution.* Sheffield: ScHARR.

NHS Executive (1998) *Nurse Consultants.* HSC 1998/161. Leeds: NHS Executive.

NHS Management Executive (1991) *Junior Doctors: The New Deal.* London: NHSME.

NHS Modernisation Agency (2003) *New Ways of Working*. www.modern.nhs.uk/scripts/ default.asp?site_id=47 (accessed 17 April 2005). See also www.modern.nhs.uk/ newwaysofworking/NWWSummer.pdf.

National Institute for Clinical Excellence (2000) *Guidance on Implantable Cardio-verter Defibrillators for Arrhythmias*. Technology Appraisal Guidance Number 11. www.nice.org.uk/Docref.asp?d=10239 (accessed 14 April 2005).

National Institute for Clinical Excellence (2002) *Final Appraisal Determination: Drugs for Early Thrombolysis in the Treatment of Acute Myocardial Infarction*. www.nice.org.uk/ page.aspx?o=36672 (accessed 14 April 2005).

National Primary Care Research and Development Centre, University of Manchester (1999) *A Bibliography of Skill Mix in Primary Care – The Sequel*. Manchester: NPRCD.

Norton L (2000) The role of specialist nurse in weaning patients from mechanical ventilation and the development of a nurse-led approach. *Nursing in Critical Care* **5**(5): 220–227.

Nursing and Midwifery Council (2004) *NMC Questionnaire on the Proposed Framework for the Standard for Post-registration Nursing*. London: NMC.

Quinn T (1998) Early experience of nurse-led elective DC cardioversion. *Nursing in Critical Care* **3**(2): 59–62.

Quinn T, Allen TF, Thompson DR, Pawelec J and Boyle RM (1999) Identification of patients suitable for direct admission to a coronary care unit by ambulance para-medics. *Pre-hospital Immediate Care* **3**: 126–130.

Raftery J, Yao G, Murchie P, Campbell N and Lewis DM (2005) Cost-effectiveness of nurse led secondary prevention clinics for coronary heart disease in primary care: follow up of a randomized controlled trial. *British Medical Journal* **330**: 707.

Read S (1998) Exploring new roles in nursing: a researcher's perspective. In: Fulbrook P and Rolfe G (eds). *Perspectives on Advanced Nursing*. Oxford: Butterworth Heinemann.

Read S, Lloyd Jones M, Collins K, McDonnell A, Jones R, Doyal L *et al.* (1999) *Exploring New Roles in Practice: Implications of Developments within Clinical Teams* (ENRiP). Executive Summary Sheffield University: ScHARR.

Richardson A and Cunliffe L (2003) New horizons: the motives, diversity and future of 'nurse-led' care. *Journal of Nursing Management* **11**(2): 80–84.

Roberts-Davis M and Read S (2001) Clinical role clarification: using the Delphi method to establish similarities and differences between nurse practitioners and clinical nurse specialists. *Journal of Clinical Nursing* **10**: 33–43.

Rolfe G and Fulbrook P (1998) *Advanced Nursing Practice*. London: Butterworth-Heinemann.

Rosen R and Mountford L (2002) Developing and supporting extended nursing roles: the challenges of NHS walk-in centres. *Journal of Advanced Nursing* **39**(3): 241–248.

Royal College of Nursing (1988) *Specialties in Nursing*. London: RCN.

Royal College of Nursing (2004) *Nurse Practitioners – An RCN Guide to Nurse Practitioner Roles, Competencies and Programme Accreditation*. London: RCN.

Royal College of Surgeons of England (1999) *Assistants in Surgical Practice: A Discussion Document*. London: RCS.

Rushforth H and Glasper A (1999) Implications of nursing role and expansion for professional practice. *British Journal of Nursing* **8**(22): 1507–1513.

Salussolia M (1997) Is advanced nursing practice a post or person? *British Journal of Nursing* **6**(18): 928–933.

Scholes J, Furlong S and Vaughan B (1999) New roles in practice: charting three typologies of role innovation. *Nursing in Critical Care* **4**(6): 268–275.

Shah M and Shah N (2004) Should nurses not do nursing? *British Medical Journal* **329**: 892–894.

Smallwood A (2004) Nurse-initiated thrombolysis: a systematic review of the literature. *Nursing in Critical Care* **9**(1): 4–12.

Strömberg A (2002) Educating nurses and patients to manage heart failure. *European Journal of Cardiovascular Nursing* **1**(1): 33–40.

Tagney J (2004) Can nurses in cardiology areas prepare patients for implantable cardioverter defibrillator implant and life at home? *Nursing in Critical Care* **9**(3): 104–114.

Tagney J, James J and Albarran JW (2003) Exploring the patient's experiences of learning to live with an implantable cardioverter defibrillator (ICD) from one UK centre – a qualitative study. *European Journal of Cardiovascular Nursing* **2**(3): 195–203.

Thompson DR and Stewart S (2002) Nurse-directed services: how can they be made more effective? *European Journal of Cardiovascular Nursing* **1**(1): 7–10.

Thompson DR and Watson R (2005) The state of nursing in the United Kingdom. *Journal of Clinical Nursing* **14**: 1039–1040.

Tripp C, Screaton M, Sharples L, Kearsley N and Caine N (2002) Development and evaluation of the critical care practitioner role. *Nursing in Critical Care* **7**(5): 227–234.

United Kingdom Central Council (1990) *Post Registration Education and Practice Project*. London: UKCC.

United Kingdom Central Council (1992a) *The Scope of Professional Practice*. London: UKCC.

United Kingdom Central Council (1992b) *The Code of Professional Conduct*. London: UKCC.

United Kingdom Central Council (1994) *The Future of Professional Practice – The Council's Standards for Education and Practice Following Registration*. London: UKCC.

United Kingdom Central Council (1998) *Report on Higher Level Practice* (Specialist Practice Project – Phase II). London: UKCC.

Waller S (1998) Higher level practice in nursing: a prerequisite for nurse consultants? *Hospital Medicine* **59**(10): 816–817.

West JA, Miller NH, Parker KM, Senneca D, Ghandour G, Clark M *et al.* (1997) A comprehensive management system for heart failure improves clinical outcomes and reduces medical resource utilization. *American Journal of Cardiology* **79**: 58–63.

Wiggens L (1998) Specialist practice and the professional project for nursing. *British Journal of Nursing* **7**(5): 266–269.

Chapter 10
Future gazing: the place for expert nursing?

Introduction

In this chapter the exploration turns to consider learning transitions that will help the profession to change to meet the challenges of the future. The pace of change is likely to be radical and rapid, and critical care leaders will need to be at the forefront influencing decisions and care provision. This will require them to be creative and sometimes courageous as they attempt to assimilate new ways of working that retain caring as the core value and ensure that nursing can retain its rightful place beside the critically sick patient and their relatives.

Leadership for the future

What futuristic concerns might face the critical care nursing experts in the future? One thing is certain: the pace of development and change will continue to push back the boundaries of critical care. If nursing is to survive, it will have to keep pace with all the challenges and transmogrify to accommodate new and diverse aspects of clinical practice. It is important to look to the future and consider the possibilities, not least so that nursing leaders might position themselves to be actively involved in the restructuring and reshaping of services.

Future gazing is a risky business. All we can know is that the future is uncertain but will certainly bring change. The rapid advancement of technology set in a context of an ageing, more informed public is set to increase the debate about what treatments can be delivered to whom and under what conditions within the funding limitations of health care provision. Five key issues have been identified as being instrumental in reshaping critical care provision within the next two decades. They are:

- advances in biotechnology;
- moral and ethical health care and economics of provision;
- hospitals as intensive care units;

- the emergence of new professions;
- information technology and the place of critical care nursing.

Advances in biotechnology

Stem cell research is leading to some significant advances in biotechnology. Indeed it has been said to hold 'the greatest potential for the alleviation of suffering since the introduction of antibiotics' (Robinson, 2005). Researchers in the field suggest that stem cell therapy may eventually be used for more effective treatment of disease. In some instances it has even been proposed as a cure for heart disease, diabetes, burns and spinal cord injuries, as well as Parkinson's disease, multiple sclerosis and certain types of cancer (National Institutes for Health, 2000). However, progress in technology is fraught with challenging ethical and political debates, and the current rise in religious fundamentalism alongside an anti-technology backlash (founded on the anti-globalisation capitalism agenda) may significantly impact upon progress.[1]

Despite scientists in Seoul creating the first customised human embryonic stem cell to treat injured or sick patients in the laboratory (June 2005), this method of tissue replacement as treatment for disease in patients is many years away from being tested and in therapeutic use (Neergaard, 2005). Until such treatments are in widespread therapeutic use, we can only speculate on the impact on the profile of patients who will be treated in critical care environments and the type of system support they may require. Stem cell treatment is but one of a series of therapies that are set to revolutionise health care. For example, in the more distant future, there is the possibility of smart bacteria, linked together by infrared, to make sophisticated self-organising circuits that target specific diseased cells or infected organs (Pearson, 2005).

As technology advances and the capacity to sustain life is increased, the promise of 'revolutionary therapies' to reverse conditions otherwise deemed hopeless may result in patients enduring life support and invasive therapies which may seem 'a violation of the human spirit' (Hickey, 1996: 350). To stand beside the patient and advocate on their behalf whilst supporting relatives through complex and difficult decisions is the place in which nurses should find themselves to guard against the 'current mutation of the nursing role and the increasing loss of the foundational place in the bedside delivery of total patient care' (Bradshaw, 2000: 328).

---

[1] For example, research using human embryo stem cells has been authorised in the UK but was initially halted in the US by President Bush. In 2001, Bush decided that this research could resume but only using existing lines of stem cells. However, it was estimated that this stock was gradually degrading and that by May 2005 they would all be useless for research (Robinson, 2005). In the same month, a federal bill was passed that allowed for funded research on embryonic stem cells extracted from surplus embryos in fertility clinics. President Bush remains resolutely opposed to such usage (State of the Union Speech, 2006).

Moral and ethical health care and economics of provision

Increasingly, ethical and moral arguments will be heard in the public arena. Less audible will be the discussions held by risk-aversive stakeholders. With growing public power in directing health care provision, the professions (or what remains of them) will need to become more inclusive and transparent in involving the client in the decision-making process about treatment options. However, although a welcome advance, the impact of public ethical and moral debate with decisions finalised in the courts can potentially lead to paralysis or over-defensive practice.[2] Clinical leaders have to exercise great courage, fortitude and commitment to follow through issues, especially in controversial areas where they believe they are acting in the best interests of the patient (RCN Institute, 2002). Once again it is important for the voice of critical care nursing to be heard to influence and champion the cause of the patient. But the specialists who assume such roles will need to be equipped with different types of knowledge that are drawn from philosophical, ethical, moral and legal reasoning to scaffold their clinical understanding of critical care.

Hospitals as intensive care units

As more patients are treated in the community, hospitals might well become centres that treat patients with the highest levels of dependency requiring the most sophisticated or experimental technology to support them (Hickey, 1996). Three types of provision will become clearer: hospital provision for emergency, urgent and critical care; primary care where the bulk of provision will be provided, including the management of long-term conditions (LTCs), in community facilities[3] (and possibly in the future specific emergency and acute care needs); and finally planned surgery or intervention, provided by the private health care sector that is either commissioned by the health service or funded by private insurance (DH, 2000). Although this type of provision seems logical,

---

[2] An example is the recent case of Charlotte Wyatt. Charlotte was born three months premature and weighed a pound. She has spent all her life in hospital requiring oxygen therapy and enteral hyperalimentation (tube feeding). She has been resuscitated three times and her doctors went to the courts to request that if she arrested again they would not need to aggressively resuscitate her, claiming this was in Charlotte's best interests (based on quality of life, assumptions about the longevity of her life and apparent pain and discomfort of the baby). Her parents, on religious grounds, claimed that Charlotte should be given every treatment option to enable her to continue her 'fight for life'. Two doctors were prepared to perform an elective tracheotomy and start ventilation if she stopped breathing, but the judge Mr Justice Hedley, ruled that if Charlotte had another respiratory arrest it was in her best interests not to be revived. The judge concluded this was the most compassionate route for the baby although recognising the agony of the parents (Mullins, 2005).

[3] The current plan is to reduce emergency bed days by 5% in 2008 through the provision of improved care in the community and primary care settings (NaTPaCT, 2005a).

it raises concern for the patients who are discharged from hospitals. Some may be managed by the new LTC teams (NatPaCT, 2005b), but other patients with acute onset needs may find they require intermediate or step-down care to facilitate their transition from a highly dependent facility into self-care and independence, which are not covered by the LTC care pathways. Whether critical care nurses provide this service to ensure continuity and build on the relationships they have established whilst in the units is an issue that is yet to be resolved, but one on which they will need to assert their position.

Currently, the demand for critical care outreach to provide a 24-hour, 7-day-a-week service has already placed a burden on staff in critical care units (Adams, 2004) and indicates a shift towards an increasingly dependent hospitalised patient population. The National Enquiry into Patient Outcomes and Death (NCEPOD, 2005) indicated that the outreach services should be adopted in all Trusts. In 2005, 44% of acute hospitals did not provide an outreach service (ibid.) However, the prediction is that critical care provision will be the universal standard throughout the hospital in the future. If this is to be the case, then more than outreach will be required to meet the changing profile and dependency of hospitalised patients. This has significant implications for the pre-registration curriculum, with calls for a fifth branch in the register to be implemented as soon as possible: one that focuses on the needs of patients who require acute and critical adult nursing (Scholes *et al.*, 2004). Curriculum content needs to shift to address far more physiology, biological science, and information technology care for patients requiring invasive and technological support, and this needs to be blended with a depth of understanding to enable nurses to deal with the ethical, moral and legal context in which they practise. This will require an honest acceptance that this field of nursing is not about 'health care' but 'illness care' (Hickey, 1996: 352) and that the nurse's place is to be beside those who suffer. The nurse's role is to: alleviate suffering (Eriksson, 1995); champion the cause of the vulnerable; and act as a catalyst to enhance imaginative and creative approaches to the provision of care within the critical care setting but also in the intermediate care stage and follow-up. However, within the current political climate that is setting the trajectory for workforce reconfiguration, this will require courageous nursing leadership and assertive, proactive interventions to assure that nursing retains its privileged position beside the patient (Benner and Wrubel, 1989).

The emergence of new professions

The recruitment and retention crisis seems to be a perennial problem. To provide the type of care outlined above will necessitate working differently. The current trend towards providing services by anyone who is deemed competent to provide them has been a powerful way to break down traditional professional boundaries and re-engineer the workforce. However, the medium of competency assessment, assurance and risk management might well prove too limited as care provision becomes more technically and ethically complex. What the competence agenda has successfully achieved is the creation of different types of practitioner who fulfil necessary health care roles but outside any philosophical or conceptual framework of care. The agenda is explicitly about organisational or workforce systems for re-engineering and restructuring (or modernising) the health service (NaPaCT, 2005b). It deliberately runs counter to any professional ethic and is justified on the grounds of breaking down boundaries and drawing individuals out of their professional silos. Although a short-term solution to address the skills shortfall, it is predicted that this strategy will fall short of public expectation and require radical review. As indicated in the next section, the prediction is that the public will call for the restoration of professional codes of conduct for all those involved in direct patient care and will seek assurance that these new professional bodies have greater control over its membership. The second driver will be the acknowledgement that enabling individuals to enter a profession, in the longer term, provides for a more satisfying career and ultimately results in greater retention.

Information technology and the place of nursing in future critical care provision

Close interaction with the critically ill patient and their family is essential to form apposite clinical judgements. In a highly technical environment it is ever more important that we can clarify what the nursing presence actually brings to the well-being of the critically ill patient. This fundamental relationship needs to be strongly defended in any debates about reshaping the provision of critical care services and re-engineering clinical roles. This has relevance for the future on two counts: first, patient monitoring, and secondly the increasing capacity of artificial intelligence to support clinical decision making.

Futurists have suggested that monitoring equipment, telemedicine and other forms of electronic surveillance will mean that expert critical care nurses might be called upon to monitor patients from a distance through these media. Benner's work indicates that this would not allow for the crucial elements of interaction which inform wise ethical and clinical judgements (Benner *et al.*, 1999).

Secondly, the increased use of artificial intelligence to support decision making might seem a favourable solution to enable less experienced or differently qualified carers to look after the critically ill. However, it is fraught with limitations, not least of which is the fact that programmed responses are more likely to deal with the technical, investigative or medical intervention to address a change in condition, but would not necessarily address the implications for nursing action.

Although these treatment options seem the stuff of science fiction, they might soon become science fact. If you consider the advancements in critical care provision in the past 25 years, and if the rate of development and progress increases at the same pace, the age, type and severity of illness that can be considered reversible with new treatments present nurses with new challenges as they seek to preserve the dignity, self-respect and comfort of the patients in their care. Distant surveillance, with smart wires and machines, and computers that create smart environments that act as sensors and communicate and change parameters according to findings are a possibility in the future. Consider the role of the commercial pilot who now monitors the computer screens and is only required to use their skills to take off and land the aircraft (or to respond in an emergency): their presence on the flight deck is mainly to allay the public's fears, as technically the plane could fly without them.

Is it possible that such equipment could be put to use in critical care environments where computers monitor other computers that calibrate and control the machines that support the patient? And, if this was the case, to what extent would there be defaults in such complex systems that would allow for an 'undo button' or delay (Steliaros, 2005)? Would these banks of visual display units be monitored by fewer, differently trained staff, there mainly to respond in an emergency or to provide intubation and weaning? This might go some way towards addressing the shortfall in available staff. However, the use of such equipment raises important questions as to where the accountability might lie: with the systems designer, the manufacturer, or the nurse in surveillance?

This scenario takes no account of the importance of human presence and the therapeutic quality of being beside a patient through their sickness. This might not be paramount in the mind of a systems designer, especially if they considered that this place could be taken by a relative with technical support and advice from a distantly located critical care adviser. This may seem ludicrous as critical care nurses intuitively know, understand and trust the power of their presence beside the patient to provide relief from the suffering of injury or iatrogenic and/or natural disease. They know how to use their therapeutic presence, but also recognise when to therapeutically absent themselves, leaving the patient to rest but remaining in close proximity and maintaining a high state of vigilance to monitor for any changes and respond immediately (Scholes and Moore, 1997). They also know of the suffering, fear and isolation of the relatives who sit beside those they love who are in desperate ill health. To imagine distancing oneself from the patient and relatives to adopt a displaced position of surveillance and offering remote intervention suggests a world where nursing no longer exists.

These issues might seem like a flight of fancy and vaguely ridiculous, but to what extent have the advanced machines that we use today actually caused greater distance between the patient and the nurse? Unless we can provide a coherent body of evidence that can justify the case for keeping nurses at the bedside of the critically ill, critical care nursing faces a very uncertain future. But of greatest concern is where this might leave the critically ill patient and their relatives if there is no nurse beside them to bring comfort in their suffering.

Future predictions on trends and drivers for critical care provision

If trends are to shift in the direction predicted above, I think a number of things might happen (based on other societal trends) that shape the way new technologies and research that influence future critical care provision are commissioned, governed and delivered. They are:

- the impact of rising fundamentalism and conservatism;
- funding for science and technology;
- public involvement;
- the (re)emergence of revered intellectuals and professionals;
- the restoration of trust in the new professions.

The rise of fundamentalism and conservatism

This might result in the rejection of advanced technology or increased suspicion about science and technology, temporarily suspending or permanently crushing potential advances in science on religious, political or social grounds. This could result in a prolonged period of intellectual and technological recession that results in the stasis (if not regression) of such developments in favour or alternative, natural treatments. However, this might give rise to tensions between those advocating the continued use of existing treatments to support life and those who feel that the quality of life agenda should be paramount.

Funding for science and technology moves into the private sector

Funding may move away from the Government into the private sector, which holds a profit motive for developments (Pearson, 2005). This might evoke a new debate about access to health technologies that is universal (globally) and not confined to wealthy societies. Ultimately, the companies or conglomerates responsible for the new technologies might choose to become providers of certain services or packages of critical care, for specific patient pathways. They may train their staff differently, to work exclusively with their products in a niche market that only the very rich can buy. Shifting such provision into the market-for-profit sector would mean that public accountability for the safe delivery of health care is driven by an agenda to please shareholders.[4]

Furthermore, if funding for leading-edge research is driven into the private sector, there might be undue pressure for success and reduction in the tolerance for failure or at least in open discussion about failure. This is risky as it reduces the ability to learn from mistakes, and increases the predisposition

---

[4] It is recognised that shareholders have little stomach for a public scandal. This might result in a private company having to be more public and transparent about the services they provide, even if they are less transparent about their research and development agenda.

towards risk aversion and conservatism that can ultimately stifle innovation (Steliaros, 2005).

Public involvement

Cost, moral argument and access to treatment (e.g. stage of illness, age, the extent to which the individual is considered 'culpable' through lifestyle choices for having increased the chances of disease, the ability to pay or sub-sidise treatment costs) are all issues that will be set by the requisite policies, guidelines and implementation protocols but will be heavily influenced by societal views if they are to find acceptance (Steliaros, 2005).

With such rapid advancement, critical decisions have to be made. Steerage and representation are the bywords used by politicians to satisfy themselves that they have achieved some degree of public satisfaction that they have con-trol or influence on the way technology is advancing. MORI opinion polls and the continued use of focus groups can only sample the public mood and the increasing concern that 'consultation' has been cynically manipulated to pro-vide *policy-based evidence,* as opposed to evidence-based policy (Brown, 2001), within the 'denoncracy' at Number 10 (Seldon, 2004: 692).[5] Public disaffection will result in a radical shift in direction. For example, steering groups with a macro perspective on whole system development (not single projects) will come into being, forming consultative panels comprising lay representatives supported by experts (Steliaros, 2005). These will still need to be reflexively managed to allay public fears that the meta organisation will not ultimately gain power and impose tyrannical rule (as depicted in so many science fiction films).

All those involved in leading edge science can promise is greater con-sultation with the press, the public and politicians along with the promise to release information so that these discussions can be informed. But it will need to be a careful juggling act to balance 'adequate' consultation and the elusive pursuit of consensus which could ultimately lead to paralysis.

The consequences of this could be far reaching. For example, if the current trend for public involvement extends to global discussions over the introduc-tion of the most significant health care technologies that might affect humanity, how might this affect leading edge technology and research? The risk would be that the global consultative process would create a bureaucratic juggernaut of such power that total stasis would be achieved. As an outcome, funding and the delivery of such projects would be driven underground, with the more con-troversial yet promising health care technologies being funded by the criminal underworld who envisage enormous profit in the longer term (Pearson, 2005).

---

[5] The quotes by Brown (2001) and Seldon (2004) were originally used by Watson and Bowden (2005) in their occasional paper: 'The Turtle and the Fruit Fly: New Labour and UK Higher Edu-cation' and have been translated for use into the context of future critical care provision.

When, or if, revolutionary health care technologies emerge from research and development funded (and possibly tested) via criminal means and if they eventually reach the public market, what do we do with the new technologies they have created, especially if the public insist on their widespread availability?

The (re)emergence of revered intellectuals and professionals

In light of these changes it is predicted that the anti-intellectual and anti-professional lobby that gained ground in the 1980s will lose its strength as disempowered stakeholders seek professional champions for their cause. This will lead to a new generation of intellectual and professional experts who are publicly accountable but are called upon to advise and harness opinion to drive forward ethical yet technically advanced research.

It is predicted that such a process will be hastened by the public who seek assurance that health is being provided by carers who work to a professional ethic (and not just on the basis of competence assessment) that ensures greater accountability, exacting standards of quality control and decisive action when those standards are not realised. In response to this the professional bodies will have to shift away from self-evaluation of competence and fitness for practice and exert far greater control over their membership.

It is predicted that there will be regrouping and reformation as old professions form new ones that blur traditional role boundaries and blend different knowledge bases and skills. They will work in specialist collectives and/or teams bound by a professional ethic and duty of care providing specialised services. Each member of the collective will understand how they make a contribution within their service and how this is articulated with the services provided by other colleagues within their team. This will result in the reconfiguration of the macro agencies providing health and social care that allows for a more logical flow and intersection of services.

The limitations of patient pathways will be recognised as deficient by the public who will demand the restoration of more individualised approaches to meeting patient need. To meet these new needs, agencies, not the professionals who work within them, will need to be re-engineered. This will herald the demise of the project manager and a backlash against managerialism. The service might then find itself at a crossroads, either replacing 'the old style manager' with technicians or technologists or seeking to divert this money to fund front-line clinicians working alongside the clients. Hope over experience leads to the prediction that more clinicians will be funded to provide front-line services. This enables a new era of trust in which the patient and health care professional work together in open, transparent and progressive ways.

The restoration of public trust in the new professions

The patient and their relatives trust that health care professionals will act in their best interests, and wherever possible use the latest, sometimes experimental, approaches to care for them. The health care professional assumes that they can trust the patient and their relatives, thus dissolving the static and inhibiting culture of risk-aversive practice.

Accountability for waste production and disposal

Each one of these issues will take place in a context of macro societal agendas that take account of the accountability for waste production and pollution and global risks. In the future, hospitals will be called to account for the amount of environmental pollution they create (Purchasing and Supply Agency (PASA), 2004). New systems will need to be devised for reducing greenhouse gases, and there will need to be a drive towards more power-efficient systems. Hospital waste management and wherever possible recycling need to be considered whilst at the same time ensuring there is no risk to the local community. Currently the NHS spends £11 million per annum on disposing of the rubbish it generates (a staggering 385 000 tonnes in 2003: Moore, 2005). Critical care environments contribute significantly to rubbish generation. Discussion with manufacturers to reduce the amount of packaging around equipment is one small step towards waste reduction (PASA, 2005). Simply recycling paper, cans and domestic rubbish generated by staff is a small but significant step (Moore, 2005). In the longer term, there will be a need to develop less environmentally damaging cleaning agents that combat resistant and resilient microbes. Alternatives to incineration include the use of chemicals and the extension of heat and steam treatments, and there is also irradiation. Each one is bound to evoke different sets of challenges and different lobby groups championing alternative solutions. These may seem like non-clinical issues, but it will be staff along with the public who will make these types of change happen.

Global risks

Travel, information technology and communication highways have made significant impacts upon health care provision. To the good this has enabled cultural blending and the merging of eastern and western health care practices. For the bad, this has meant that certain diseases linked with culturally defined lifestyles (e.g. obesity, heart disease and diabetes) are now spreading into new cultural communities. Rapid travel has resulted in the spread of infection, raising widespread concern for the risk of a pandemic. Viruses seem to be crossing from animals to humans and creating devastating pathophysiological responses in the host. Many patients suffering from these illnesses require critical care nursing, and staff have fallen victim to the infections. New systems to eradicate the transmission of infections between staff and patients without totally removing them from patient contact will need to be devised if staff safety is to be assured.

The risk of terrorism, bacterial warfare and conflict have to be considered when thinking about the future of critical care services and how the service might respond to such a crisis.

Security into and out of a critical care environment has become increasingly more stringent in the past decade. But consider the damage that could be done by remote devices. For example, there is the risk of a computer virus entering the hospital's system, which if minor ends up misrouting patient information and if serious results in the loss of patient data altogether. If terrorists developed a mega blip which could wipe out micro chips, the damage that could do to a critical care unit and the machinery that the computer drives is a horrifying thought. Mobile phones are not immune – proof of a concept virus has shown that (BT, 2005) – therefore disaster planning to take account of data attack and its implications for patient care requires urgent consideration.

There are also the issues of identity theft, extortion and fraud. Identity theft to allow for travel and theft of property is a recognised problem. It is predicted that in future identity theft might be used to gain fraudulent access to health care denied to the thief because of their age, ethnicity, or past lifestyle or to gain access to prescription-only drugs. The security response has to be carefully considered to ensure that it is not so constraining that it evokes challenges over civil liberty, yet not so liberal as to expose individuals to great risk.

Once again, this sounds more to do with science fiction than science fact, but consider the investments that are being made by industry and governments to protect their IT systems from such collateral damage (BT, 2005). In the past, the greatest threat to an intensive care unit and hospital was fire or power failure. Now security, longer term independent power generation and damage-resistive buildings are part of any discussion on the commissioning of new buildings. This is no longer a matter for major disaster planning teams, but one where individuals have to take these risks seriously. The leaders of critical nursing will need to reflect on how global risks will impact upon their relative micro communities of critical care, and ensure that proposed solutions or strategies do not compromise the well-being of patients and their relatives.

Having examined some of the potential issues that face critical care nursing in the future, it is important to consider some strategies that can be used to safeguard a practitioner's positive attributes, especially in light of extreme challenge. This toolkit is of equal value to any transitioner who is making their journey towards expertise (Table 10.1).

Conclusion

The pace and dynamic of change are rapid. Critical care is at the forefront of providing new technologies for life support, and nurses experience first hand the consequences of providing leading-edge treatments for their patients. In addition, their skills are called upon to support colleagues caring for dependent patients in environments outside the traditional boundaries of the critical care

Table 10.1   A tool kit for surviving transitions.

- Trust your own intuitive processes.
- Conduct an organisational analysis – know about the context in which you work.
- Keep abreast of local, regional and national health policy issues, in particular views about nurses and their contribution to health care.
- Review your job description – it is a useful road map to guide your performance and to identify disablers such as lack of individual performance review or clinical supervision.
- Articulate and clarify your professional nursing role to colleagues, peers, patients and the public. The more often you articulate your role the more you will believe it.
- Create a supportive network of like-minded professional nurses. Recognise that not all nurses want to develop professional nursing practice.
- Keep the ambiguities of professional nursing practice in perspective; try not to take it all personally.
- Maintain a positive self-concept: it will serve to maintain your internal locus of control.
- Nurture yourself, be kind to yourself, have some 'me time'.
- Use your imagination and take risks; this involves believing in what you do and developing and growing in your role as a professional nurse.
- Use personal planning skills; know what you want to achieve and how you are going to get there.
- Cultivate supportive, collegial relationships.
- Maintain your commitment to lifelong learning: new knowledge can capture your imagination, leading to new horizons and new understandings.
- Develop measurable and achievable outcomes for each year; include an evaluation plan.
- Conduct periodic self-reflection through critical reflection with a critical companion.
- Generate a monthly activity summary: see what you have achieved; what else could you have achieved or given, for example, appropriate skill mix and patient throughput.
- Recognise the 'dose of nursing' in what you do and focus on its impact for patients and carers.

(Hixon, 1996 adapted by Norris, 2000)

environment. This means that the services that are provided within such units and the clinicians who deliver that care have to adapt and constantly refine their skills to meet the needs of patients and their relatives.

Currently macro organisational change agents (e.g. Skills for Health, the Modernisation Agency) have used tools and techniques (e.g. competence frameworks, patient care pathways) to redefine and reconfigure the workforce and re-engineer services, resulting in a somewhat passive response by the nursing profession. In the future, and through the medium of visionary clinical leaders, it is predicted that nurses (or practitioners who make up the new professions), will foster a more proactive role in determining how they can develop to best meet the needs of patients and their relatives. Thereby, pragmatic solutions envisioned within organisational systems frameworks will be replaced by clinically sensitive and genuinely patient-centred approaches to determine care provision. In this way it is hoped that more resilient services will develop that accommodate dramatic political shifts in direction, which currently create massive organisational upheaval and chaos.

Some authors (e.g. Hickey, 1996) suggest that there will be greater resilience towards significant change. Currently there seems to be no such resilience, rather an exhausted, demoralised workforce (Norris, 2000) ready to accept the new set of changes being implemented by their Trusts, insecure in the knowledge that shifts in organisational thinking will redirect funding into the latest politically motivated project. This results in a lack of consolidation of services, transient practitioners unable to consolidate their knowledge and become experts, and most importantly, a crisis in the public's confidence in the treatment they will receive whilst in health care.

Within this context it is important for nurses to regroup and refocus. If the advances in health care are set to develop at the pace promised by futurists, it is essential for this to happen. The most significant issue is to recognise, articulate and champion the need for therapeutic nursing, grounded in a knowledge base that keeps apace with new developments but is driven by the core value of bringing comfort to those who suffer, which is encapsulated by a professional ethic.

The role of the critical care nurse will change, but if future historians look back at the beginning of the 21st century and can no longer identify anything that resembles a form of practice that was once claimed to be nursing, who will they blame for the extinction? (Hickey, 1996) Nurse leaders need to learn from the profession's past learning transitions and champion the best care provision for the critically ill patient and their relatives.

This is not a clarion cry to return to the good-old, bad-old days of nursing, nor is it stated with the sole concern for professional self-interest. These are trumped-up charges levied by individuals who are driving forward their own political, organisational or managerial agendas. They may claim to be pushing forward a programme of modernisation that hinges on providing greater public accountability in meeting patient need, but they do so on the basis of never having been, even in their recent past, closely engaged in providing front-line services. It is time for nurses to stand up confidently for what they know from their everyday clinical experience: when someone is critically ill, they and their relatives need to be supported by a caring, empathic and knowledgeable professional. It is at that time that the practitioner calls themselves a nurse. Is there any real cause to call them other?

References

Adams S (2004) Plugging the gap – critical care skills are the current universal commodity. *Nursing in Critical Care* **9**(5): 195–198.

Benner P and Wrubel J (1989) *The Primacy of Caring: Stress and Coping in Health and Illness*. Menlo Park, CA: Addison Wesley.

Benner P, Hooper Kyriakidis P and Stannard D (1999) *Clinical Wisdom and Interventions in Critical Care. A Thinking in Action Approach*. Philadelphia: WB Saunders.

Bradshaw A (2000) Editorial, Special Issue: Competence. *Journal of Clinical Nursing* **9**(3): 319–329.

Brown R (2001) *Evidence Based Policy or Policy Based Evidence*. City University Teaching and Learning Monograph Series (December). London: City University.

British Telecommunications (2005) Security in the spot light. Looking ahead to future threats. www.btglobalservices.com/business/global/en/business/business_zone/issue_02/security_spotlight.html (accessed 7 September 2005).

Department of Health (2000) *The NHS Plan*. London: DH.

Eriksson K (1995) *Det Lidende Menneske* [The suffering human being]. Copenhagen: Munsgaard.

Hickey J (1996) Advanced nursing practice: moving into the 21st century in practice, education and research. In Hickey J, Ouimette RM and Venegoni S (eds). *Advanced Practice Nursing: Changing Roles and Clinical Applications*. Philadelphia: Lippincott Williams & Wilkins: 350–360.

Hixon M (1996) Professional development: socialisation in advanced practice nursing. In Hickey J, Ouimette RM and Venegoni S (eds). *Advanced Practice Nursing: Changing Roles and Clinical Applications*. Philadelphia: Lippincott Williams & Wilkins: 33–53.

Moore A (2005) Going green. *Nursing Standard* **19**(31): 24–26.

Mullins M (2005) The case of Charlotte Wyatt. Licc London Institute for Contemporary Christianity. Connecting with Culture. www.licc.org.uk/culture/the-case-of-charlotte-wyatt (accessed 6 May 2005).

National Enquiry into Patient Outcomes and Death (2005) *An Acute Problem?* London: NCEPOD.

National Institutes for Health (2000) NIH publishes final guidelines for stem cell research. National Institutes for Health, 23 August 2000 (available from www.nih.gov/news/pr/aug2000/od-23.htm).

National Primary and Care Trusts Development Programme (2005a) Supporting patients with long term conditions. Available from www.natpact.nhs.uk/cms/2.php.

National Primary and Care Trusts Development Programme (2005b) Workforce change in long term conditions programme. www.natpact.nhs.uk/cms/393.php.

Neergaard L (2005) Korean Scientists clone stem cells. *Fosters News* at: www.fosters.com/apps/pbcs.dll/article?AID=/20050602/NEWS40/105190165 (accessed 6 June 2005).

Norris M (2000) Contextual factors that enable or disable nurses' professional practice. Unpublished DPhil Thesis, University of Sussex.

Pearson I (2005) Presentation by Ian Pearson, BT Futurist To: EPSRC/ESRC Workshop on the policy implications and societal impacts of new technologies. 1st March 2005, London.

Purchasing and Supply Agency (2004) Towards sustainability – Taking a closer look 2003/4, Case studies, Total waste management. www.pasa.nhs.uk/sustainabledevelopment/2004/casestudies/wastemanagement.htm (accessed 8 June 2005).

Purchasing and Supply Agency (2005) Total waste management services. Packaging and supply initiatives. NHS Sustainable Development and Environmental Purchasing and Supply Forum. Available from www.pasa.nhs.uk/sustainabledevelopment/environment/proc.stm. Updated 8 June 2005.

Robinson B (2005) Stem cell research. All sides to the dispute at http://www.religioustolerance.org/res_stem.htm (accessed 6 May 2005).

Royal College of Nursing Institute (2002) *Expertise in Practice Project: Exploring Expertise.* London: RCN.

Scholes J and Moore M (1997) *Making a Difference: the Way in which the Nurse Interacts with the Critical Care Environment and Uses Herself as a Therapeutic Tool.* ITU NDU Occasional Paper Series Number 2 (University of Brighton) [ISBN 1 87196679 5].

Scholes J, Freeman F, Gray M, Wallis B, Robinson D, Matthews-Smith G and Miller C (2004) Evaluation of Nurse Education Partnerships. Available from: www.brighton.ac.uk/inam/research/projects/partnerships_report.pdf.

Seldon A (2004) *Blair.* London: Free Press.

State of the Union Speech (2006) www.whitehouse.gov/stateoftheunion/2006/index.html (accessed 24 April 2006).

Steliaros R (2005) Policy implications and societal impacts of new technologies. EPSRC/ESRC Workshop on the policy implications and societal impacts of new technologies. London.

Watson D and Bowden R (2005) The turtle and the fruit fly: New Labour and UK Higher education 2001–2005. Education Research Centre Occasional Paper. Brighton: ERC, University of Brighton.

Index